DRINK UP!

How Ten Days Ended a Lifetime of Addiction

KATHLEEN S.

authorHOUSE®

AuthorHouse™
1663 Liberty Drive
Bloomington, IN 47403
www.authorhouse.com
Phone: 1-800-839-8640

First published by AuthorHouse 11/19/2010

ISBN: 978-1-4567-1053-8 (sc)
ISBN: 978-1-4567-1054-5 (e)

Library of Congress Control Number: 2010917503

Printed in the United States of America

Book Cover Art by John Browning

CONTENTS

Runnin' hot,
Runnin' cold,
I was running into overload,
It was extreme.
New Attitude
Jon Gilutin, Bunny Hull, Sharon Terea Robinson

PROLOGUE

Alcohol is killing me. But it doesn't make me high; there is no buzz. My sole objective in using is to go from consciousness to unconsciousness in the fastest time possible. Alcohol oozes out of my pores, silently and not so silently destroying my life.

I spend the time between binges regretting. Recovering from the poison that renders my movements slow and clumsy; that turns my once sharp brain into a pile of rubble. That emotionally fills me with guilt, shame, self-loathing.

My binges are triggered by a variety of things. By *everything*. Insomnia. An episode of low self-esteem. Anxiety. Having a bad day. Having a great day.

Even my triggers have triggers.

I am a 56-year-old woman who knows what alcohol is doing to me. Who knows I have to give it up. Yet, even after the deaths of my father from alcohol, my brother Mike from a heroin overdose in his 40s, my brother Gary from alcohol poisoning in *his* 40s, I can't do it.

I *can't* do it…

I'm rapidly losing whatever hold I still have on life. In fact, given my genetics, family history, and past behavior patterns, I'm already living on borrowed time.

> **I took it so high, so low,**
> **So low,**
> **There was no where to go**
> **Like a bad dream**
> *New Attitude*
> Jon Gilutin, Bunny Hull, Sharon Terea Robinson

PART 1
BEFORE

I've been working on my drinking career for a long time now, going from a glass or two of wine on weekends to the same quantity every night. To two, three glasses. Bigger glasses. A full bottle. To vodka, because you can't smell it. As if.

Working my way from drinking socially with people, to drinking *before* I drink socially with people so they won't know how much I need to make it through the night. To predrinking so much I can no longer leave the house once I start.

I've evolved into a binge drinker, each binge lasting from one to three days, with one to three weeks in between. Each day I drink a fifth of vodka, gin or tequila. Or more. During my binges I lie alone in my guest bedroom. Drink until I pass out. Come to occasionally to maybe eat something. And to drink more. I do this until I've drunk so much the alcohol no longer makes me unconscious.

This is the signal that my binge is over.

I stop drinking for a day or two, swear I'll never do it again. Two days later I'm planning my next binge. It's what gets me through my days.

During my sober moments I'm aware of how empty—no—how desolate my life has become. How extreme my circumstances are. That I could soon end up just like my brothers.

Dead.

I've tried so many ways to stop drinking, looking for that magic bullet, the one that will cure me forever.

I attended a 90-day women's intensive outpatient program that consisted mostly of group therapy and support. I was sober for two years, but I always thought about booze, continued to have cravings, even when I wasn't drinking.

I've been to a naturopath.

I've had acupuncture treatments.

I take antidepressants.

I've taken Antabuse.

I take multiple vitamin and mineral supplements.

I've even been to a hypnotist.

I had an intervention by two of my best friends.

My friends—the few who know I have a drinking problem—urged me to go into rehab. One of my friends has been to a 30-day treatment program where she has beaten her marijuana addiction. I researched it and other programs. They're expensive, they last a long time (28-90 days, some six months to a year), and the treatment methods didn't appeal to my practical nature.

AA meetings don't appeal to me either. I don't like having to say I'm an alcoholic, present tense, every time I talk. I don't like the idea of turning my life over to a higher power, to admit I'm powerless.

I went to a counselor trained in treating addiction. She listened to my account of growing up in a violently alcoholic home and diagnosed me as having Post Traumatic Stress Disorder. And alcoholism. She urged me to go to AA meetings. I insisted that my drinking was merely a symptom of my underlying condition, and when I cured the PTSD, my alcoholism would be cured too.

I worked on it—my PTSD. I was able to lose a lot of my anger—but it didn't stop my drinking.

The radio advertisements for Schick Shadel Hospital appealed to me:

"We have the highest success rate of any alcohol program in the country—70 percent—and we're right here in your backyard."

"Give us 10 days, and we'll give you back your life."

I asked my counselor about Schick Shadel. Should I go there?

"No!" she said, quite adamantly. The Hospital's treatment philosophy evidently clashed with hers.

At that point I didn't question her further and put Schick Shadel out of my mind. But then I stopped seeing her, continued binging. Damaging my relationships with family and friends. Poisoning my body, my mind. My soul.

My past few binges last longer, occur more frequently, and are scarier. I'm sicker, drunker. Falling-down drunker. Injuring myself drunker. I know I cannot continue to drink.

The last time I used vodka I mixed it with Kahlua and snacked on almonds (about a pound from one of those big five-pounders from Costco). I've never been allergic to any one of those things, but the next thing I knew, I was in the emergency room with severe allergy symptoms: eyes swollen shut, nose like a block of concrete, labored breathing.

"Anaphylactic shock!" yelled the triage nurse.

I was rushed to a bed, surrounded by medical personnel who took my vital signs, administered drugs to counter my shock, took my medical history. I didn't tell them what I had consumed in addition to the nuts because my husband, Gary, was in the room with me and I didn't want him to know.

I can't believe they couldn't smell it, didn't ask me if I had been drinking.

But they didn't.

And I literally didn't know if the medicine they gave me would cure or kill me.

Obviously, I lived. And mostly switched to gin. And never again ate nuts while drinking.

My habit is life threatening. Sooner rather than later, drinking will kill me.

TWO MONTHS PRIOR

I research Schick Shadel Hospital on the Internet, despite my counselor's reservations. Summoning all my nerve, I call the hospital and Dave, the admissions director, explains the treatment program. In addition to detox (if necessary), it consists of five counter-conditioning treatments, which "will make you nauseous and hate alcohol," and four sedation interviews using a drug similar to sodium pentathol that "will get to the subconscious reasons you drink, will plant alcohol aversion suggestions, and can cut down on months of therapy."

I don't like the part about getting nauseous ("Nobody does," says Dave). But I do like the part about the sedation interviews. I want to learn all I can about my drinking. I like the idea of "talking" to my subconscious.

"We also use treatment modalities other programs offer: group therapy, one-on-one counseling, lectures, videos, affirmations, nutrition counseling, and relaxation treatments. You can come in any time you want, and treatment ends ten days later, after detox if necessary."

The program is not cheap, but it's less expensive than the other ones I've looked at. And I really like that ten days means I only have to miss one week of work if I come in on Friday. I ask Dave to check my insurance coverage.

This is such a huge step for me—it means exposing my problem to my whole family. It means potential exposure to my employer through my insurance. I am so not ready to publicly come out of the alcohol closet. And Gary has a new job—will it get around that his wife is a lush?

Dave lets me know that most of the program will be covered with our insurance policies.

I have no more excuses.

I tell Gary about the program. In fact, as I'm recovering from my next three binges, I promise him either that I have signed up, or will sign up as soon it's convenient. When I get time off from work, when I don't have to help my friend through surgery, after my trip to the East Coast. I plan on doing it—I do!

Just not today...

THE SATURDAY BEFORE

I come to hung over—again. Feeling like crap—again. Hating myself, ashamed. The usual.

This morning, I know I can't put it off any longer. I make the call to Schick Shadel, planning to arrive Thursday evening to begin therapy Friday morning.

I can bring a computer and cell phone.

My husband and daughter share my apprehension about the type of treatment. Nevertheless, they're proud of me, relieved. And a little confused about what to say. We've never talked about my drinking all that much.

I tell my best friend, Lynn, who also lives here in the Pacific Northwest. I have known her since the fourth grade—nearly 50 years now. We grew up together in New Jersey. Lynn and her significant other were responsible for my intervention. She too is a little nervous about the type of treatment, but she's also happy I'm doing something.

After a lot of thought about what to say, I call my boss, tell her I've got some medical issues that need attention, that I'll be out for almost two weeks. She is wonderful, caring. Genuinely concerned for me and my health, having just gone through breast cancer. I feel guilty at first, thinking her illness was life threatening while mine…

And I have to remind myself that mine has become life threatening too.

She wishes me well. Tells me not to worry about work.

I'm really gonna do it.

Shit…

THE SUNDAY BEFORE

My Irish Catholic father would send me and my three brothers to church each Sunday while he went down to the local "gin mill" to get his Sunday sermon.

My mother converted to Catholicism to get married but never went to mass. I think Sunday mornings were the only time she had to herself for years.

In those days, girls had to wear hats to church. We couldn't afford one, so my mother used bobby pins to clip a hanky to my head. The nuns would look at the top of my head, then into my eyes, letting me know they didn't approve. Church was not a place where I found peace.

Those were also the days when you couldn't question the dogma without risking a ruler across your knuckles. I'd always been curious—so my knuckles were a frequent target during Saturday catechism class.

I abandoned Catholicism years ago, as soon as I could. I was angry at God, wasn't even sure what the concept of god meant.

But today I feel scared and needy.

A while ago Lynn, who also abandoned her Catholic teachings, found a unique church that fit her philosophy. I attended a few times and also liked it. I surprise her by joining her at church this morning.

"Prayers of the People" is the part of the service I like best. People call out the names of people for whom they would like prayers. The minister, a woman who radiates peace and love, repeats the names and asks the reasons for the prayers. Individual concerns become the whole congregation's concerns. I find some of the spirituality, the sense of community I need today.

Today when others are asking aloud for their loved ones, I pray silently for myself:

"Please help me conquer my alcoholism."

"Please. I want to live."

Near the end of the service, two members of the congregation sing a song from the Broadway show "Into the Woods" called "You Are Not Alone." They start at the back of the church, walk slowly down the aisle toward the altar, smiling at us as they pass each pew, lifting their strong, clear voices. The words seem meant for me today, and I get goose bumps as I listen:

> Mother cannot guide you,
> Now you're on your own.
> Only me beside you,
> Still you're not alone.
>
> No one is alone,
> Truly, no one is alone.
>
> Hard to see the light now,
> Just don't let it go.
> Things will come out right now,
> We can make it so.
>
> Someone is on your side,
> No one is alone.

THE TUESDAY BEFORE

Only two more nights of freedom, so I do what every drunk does who is about to give up alcohol (again): drink. I limit the quantity to a pint of gin and a small, airplane-size bottle of brandy so I can recover over the next day and a half before rehab. I don't want to start treatment in detox.

I drink my stash and as usual, quickly bypass any high or feel-good stage, and pass out.

ADMITTING DAY

When work ends, I head home to pack, tie up loose ends. I say goodbye to my daughter, Carolyn.

I have three kids: Carolyn and two sons ages 27 and 25 who live a distance away. Carolyn, 20, attends college in the area and stops in frequently. She has seen the worst of my alcoholism as I progressed through the years to the stage I'm at now.

I briefly think about my father and how humiliated I was by him. We lived across the street from the school I attended from kindergarten through eighth grade.

After school I would often find my father lying unconscious on the front porch in full view of the kids and teachers who parked on the block. If he wasn't passed out, he'd be yelling obscenities as people went by, sometimes at the teachers.

I know I haven't humiliated my daughter that way. But I have caused her pain, worry. I apologize to her. I know she so wants me to quit drinking.

She hugs me tightly, tells me she loves me, wishes me luck.

Before checking into the Hospital, Gary and I eat dinner at our favorite place, a storefront Afghan restaurant. Tonight a sitar player strums softly as we eat. I have my favorite meal—my Last Supper: marinated rack of lamb, eggplant burta, basmati rice with raisins, Afghan bread, cucumber salad with oil, vinegar, and mint.

At dinner, we talk—really talk. We have been married 35 years, and we're really unhappy with each other these days.

For my husband, honesty is everything. Sober, I'm as honest and trustworthy as can be (except where it concerns my drinking). But when I'm drinking, there are no rules. I'm sneaky, secretive, and a *great* liar! Two totally different people.

Gary doesn't voice it—he's a very nonconfrontational person—but I know he's asking himself how many lies I've told with regard to my drinking. How can he trust me anymore? He thinks he knows both sides of me, though he really doesn't know the extent to which I'll go or have gone to protect my "secret" drinking.

But as bad as our relationship is, it's not just my alcohol abuse that's causing our problems. He shares the responsibility.

We first met when I was 20—unhealthy, skinny, neurotic. I smoked two packs of cigarettes and drank 10 cups of coffee every day. I had such low self-esteem I could barely look at people when they talked to me. Somehow, though, Gary saw something worthwhile in me. And I saw something in him I had never seen before: a kind, intelligent, mature, "normal" human being.

I hero-worshipped him, and we fell in love. I needed him so much in the early days. And he needed to be needed.

Later, after developing some self-esteem, I became less needy as I learned to stand on my own two feet. It's not that I loved him any less, I just needed him less. And that continues to threaten him.

He reacts to this by putting me down. Sometimes he does it subtly; sometimes it's pretty blatant. And it's always hurtful. Sometimes I dare to think I'm creative. When I talk about my ideas, get the nerve to share, Gary's first reaction is to laugh or to dismiss the idea without even considering it, saying: "That won't work!"

A slap in the face. That's what it feels like. A reaffirmation that I'm stupid, worthless. I can't stand it anymore. So tonight I try to plant some seeds about how bad our relationship really is. But I'm confused. Do I want to end my marriage? I hope the sedation part of the rehab program will help clarify my thinking.

It takes about a half hour to get from the restaurant to the rehab center.

It's easily recognizable by the big neon sign that reads "Schick Shadel Hospital, Dial 1-800-Craving." Subtle.

Fortunately, the hospital itself is less obvious. Nestled at the bottom of a steep hill, it's a two-story ranch-type building that looks like it started life as a small house and had wings added to it over the years.

THE ADMISSION PROCESS

Gary and I are silent as we wait for the admissions counselor. John is about 5 feet 8 inches—a young balding guy full of energy. He asks me general questions regarding my recent drinking habits. I'm embarrassed to answer these in front of my husband, but I do. If I can't be truthful now, I might as well just go home. When we finish, I ask Gary if it was too much honesty for him, if he was surprised by anything I said. He says no, but I wonder if *he's* telling the truth now.

I sign a billion papers: privacy policy papers, consent to treatment papers, insurance papers. John tells me I won't need any insurance cards or my wallet any longer, so I ask Gary to take these home with him.

John takes a Polaroid picture of me for my file; gets me a towel, pajamas, and a robe; leads us to the room. It contains a single bed, dresser, nightstand, chair, television. A door leads to a small bathroom with toilet and sink.

Gary is sent home.

Luz, my nurse, comes in to ask more questions. "When was your last drink?"

Though I answer Tuesday, she gives me a Breathalyzer test anyway (my first ever—I wonder how I've managed to avoid it until now).

"I know you've had nothing to drink, Kathleen, but we have to do this—it's all part of the admission process."

I wonder how many people lie to them about that last drink.

She asks for my medications: Effexor for depression, Trazadone for depression and sleep, TriEst for hormone replacement therapy, Lorazepam given to me by my sleep doctor for anxiety.

While I'm here, the nurses will dispense all of these, except for the Lorazepam, which they say is addictive. I won't be getting any of that.

She clips the hospital's plastic ID bracelet with the number 30685A on my wrist: 30685 for the number of patients treated before me, "A" for alcoholic.

I am wearing a hospital ID bracelet with an "A" for alcoholic.

She weighs me—165 pounds! A lot of weight for my 5-foot 5-inch frame. This is my highest weight ever—even at nine months pregnant. All that booze… She asks for a urine sample, takes my vital signs (blood pressure, temperature, pulse). Says the next day will be easy—I'll be given a physical, a relaxation treatment, orientation, and a chance to settle in. She asks many more questions, then leaves another hundred or so papers for me to complete.

I change. An aide comes in, asks me if I want to check any valuables in the safe, takes my street clothes and luggage.

It's 10 p.m. I'm alone. I've been avoiding thinking about this moment, but now the enormity of what I'm doing hits me.

And I'm scared...

Somehow the wires uncrossed,
My tables were turned,
Never knew I had
Such a lesson to learn
New Attitude
Jon Gilutin, Bunny Hull, Sharon Terea Robinson

PART 2
DURING

DAY ONE

Hospital business begins around 6 a.m. Ida, the night nurse, takes my vital signs.

"Is this your first visit with us?" she wants to know.

Wait a minute! This is a treatment center that claims a 70%+ success rate, and the nurse wants to know if this is my first time? I say these thoughts out loud, uneasy at the question. Then she reminds me that, as part of the treatment, you return for two overnight recap sessions, at 30 and 90 days after discharge.

I settle down.

Someone comes in to draw blood. She looks at my right arm. Tells me I have great veins. I laugh. I used to be told I have great legs—now, at age 56, it's great veins.

She finds one she likes, takes the blood, leaves.

Breakfast is announced at 7 a.m. over the loudspeaker:

"Good morning. Today is Friday, and breakfast is now being served in the dining room. Thank you."

I'm hungry, so I quickly head out. The hallway seems strangely empty as I make my way downstairs. Once in the dining room, I stand at the counter behind the one other patient—a tall woman with reddish blonde hair swept up in a ponytail wearing a robe identical to mine, different pajamas.

She turns to face me.

What is treatment etiquette, I'm wondering.

I manage an awkward "Good morning."

"Good morning," she says. "My name's Barbara."

"Hi, I'm Kathy," I say, shaking her hand.

The chef—a big, burly, friendly African American named Ron—politely offers me breakfast choices. I order bacon, eggs, and toast, then sit down with Barbara.

The second announcement of the day is made: **"Good morning. All patients having Duffy treatments this morning should be up and drinking liquids."**

I have no idea what a Duffy treatment means. Barbara tells me it's the name given to the counter-conditioning treatments.

Barbara's not doing Duffys – she's being given something called faradic treatments. Again, I have no idea what that means, but before I can ask, she's called for her treatment and we go our separate ways.

I decide to keep this journal faithfully, so I return to my room, close the door, and write until the next announcement:

"Good morning. The video "Recovery and the Family" will be shown in the auditorium at 8:30. All patients, except detox patients, **are required to attend."**

The announcer's voice actually lowers to a near whisper as she says: "except detox patients" as though excusing them is a secret she can't share with anyone—as she announces it over the loudspeaker!

I head down to the auditorium. Men and women patients— many carrying pink or clear plastic pitchers of water or other fluid, all dressed in two or three variations of the same pajamas and robes—sign in, as we are required to do.

None look particularly energetic. Some are actually shuffling.

There are about 20-25 people here. A lot of the male

patients sit alone on the aisle or with several seats between them and the next patient in the same row. There are two pairs of women sitting together. I sit in a row, alone, in an aisle seat.

Ten minutes into the video, I'm paged to the nurses' station.

I'm learning that the nurses' station is the center of all things at the hospital. Patients and staff alike congregate to check out treatment schedules, order special lunches, check out today's videos, lectures, and other notices. Medications and vitamins are dispensed here if you can't wait until they're brought to your room.

Time for my EKG.

By the time it's done, the video is over. I'm journaling in my room when in walks Ruby, a slightly overweight, pretty, dark-eyed woman with short, dark, teased hair and a big smile. Very enthusiastic, very positive.

She energetically shakes my hand, introduces herself as my patient advocate, hands me a huge packet of information, and explains the rules.

"This is all about you! It's all about you!"

She wants me to know I'm to be treated with dignity and respect, and she takes me through a few scenarios in which it would be appropriate for me to take action, such as staff or even other patients acting inappropriately or disrespectfully.

"This is all about you," she repeats. In fact, she says that after almost every sentence. I am thrilled, because it's never before been all about me.

After awhile, I begin saying it with her.

Ruby says other things, including: "You have to face your treatment with raw, true-grit determination." As she says this, she snarls, frowns, lowers the tone of her voice, increases the volume.

"You're not going to be feeling good in a few days, but you'll get through the program using your [snarl, frown, low loud voice] "raw, true-grit determination."

She takes me on a brief tour of the facilities. There is a small exercise room with a few aerobic machines. She shows me the patient lounges and the outside decks—the smoking area determined by whoever gets out there first and moves the ashtrays.

There's not much else to see—I've been to the auditorium and dining room.

Having indoctrinated me, she pumps my hand vigorously as she leaves me at the nurses' station with the now familiar mantra: "Remember… this is all about you."

She marches down the hall to the next patient's room, knocks loudly on the door, trilling, "Good morning! Good morning!" I wonder if she's going to tell him it's all about him too.

As soon as she leaves, I look into my folder. There's a lot of information on affirmations—suggestions for affirmations to use during the sedation interviews, links to Web sites on affirmations, permission to create your own.

I love affirmations, and I'm excited about using them here. I've used them in the past to help me with confidence issues in different areas of my life—business and personal— and they've worked.

I immediately begin working on creating my own. I know from a series of tapes I used to listen to called "The Inner Winner" by Denis Waitley that they should be in the present tense, personal, and positive.

I'm interrupted for my physical. Dr. Davis—a thin, bespeckled, gray-haired man in his 50s—introduces himself.

"Ms. S? Dr. Davis." Shakes my hand.

"It's Kathy.

"Thanks for the offer, Ms. S, but got to keep this professional."

Well okay then.

He reviews my paperwork and medications, listens to my heart and lungs, thumps my liver, tells me it's slightly enlarged. Indicates the enlargement with his thumb and forefinger. It looks to me to be about an inch. That seems more than "slightly" to me. I'm concerned.

"Don't be," he says. "It will return to normal in a few weeks once you stop drinking. I've seen people with enlarged livers this big:" he indicates with his hands what looks like about 12 inches.

THE PROGRAM IN DETAIL

Dr. Davis then describes the program. For two days in a row, you get a counter-conditioning treatment. These treatments are referred to as Duffys, which the literature says is "an ironic reference to the Duffy's Tavern theme that many drinkers are familiar with." After that, you have one every other day, for a total of five treatments.

The goal of the Duffy is to recondition you, to make you experience unpleasant effects from what is (or once was) pleasurable. The response you have to your addictive substance has been conditioned in your brain. The therapy acts to dramatically decondition those reflexes.

To prepare for treatment, you fast from solid foods from midnight until the morning treatment, which can be anywhere from 8 a.m. to noon. You are required to drink 64 ounces of fluid (PowerAde, soda, water) before each treatment.

The treatment itself is simple: Immediately upon entering the treatment room, you drink a nausea-inducing drug. Then you drink alcohol and you throw up. You throw up in the treatment room. You are taken back to your room, where you must stay for three hours. And maybe throw up some more.

During those three hours you can't watch television, use your cell phone or computer, or do anything else but think about your addiction.

And, of course, experience more nausea.

At the end of three hours, you are released, meaning you are allowed out of your room.

Then Dr. Davis explains the sedation interviews.

After the first two Duffys, every other day you have a rehabilitation (or sedation interview), for a total of four.

Their purpose is to monitor your developing counter-conditioning to alcohol, to give you and your treatment team insight into your feelings and emotions about using and recovery. It can cut therapy time down by months by getting the information from and to your subconscious.

The treatment also provides some relaxation—a break from the strenuous, stressful emetic treatments. Another objective of the interview is to provide positive suggestions to the subconscious to encourage abstinence.

He hasn't mentioned the faradic treatments Barbara told me about, so I ask.

People who can't have Duffys because of a medical condition, prior surgery, or other miscellaneous reasons have this alternate therapy. I don't fit the categories, he says, but he describes it to me anyway:

A band is placed around your non-dominant wrist, connected to a small, battery-operated neuromuscular stimulator similar to those used in physical therapy offices. The nurse operates the device to produce a distracting and uncomfortable tingling while the patient views, swishes, and spits his drink of choice.

The patient selects the level of stimulation, which can be changed at anytime. The objective is to keep the stimulation at a level that is mildly uncomfortable but not painful. And, like the Duffys, the purpose of pairing the drinks with the unpleasant stimulation is to reduce the positive attractiveness of the alcohol.

The explanations given, Dr. Davis concludes the examination. My blood and urine tests will be reviewed with me before I leave. My EKG is normal; everything is normal. I have the all clear to start my Duffy treatments tomorrow.

Lucky me...

I've had a busy morning, and now it's lunchtime. Again, great food: tuna sandwich, chips, homemade minestrone soup, fresh watermelon chunks. I sit alone at a table for eight. There are a few men scattered around the other tables. No one is talking very much right now—lost in our own thoughts.

I'm kept busy for most of the rest of the afternoon with various things: watching a relaxation video, answering more questions, journaling.

At 4:15, I leave my room to attend the mandatory lecture on relapse prevention.

RELAPSE PREVENTION

Because patients come in and out of the program at different times, all the lectures, workshops, videos, etc. are cycled to make sure everyone sees everything. Today's topic is "Relapse Prevention".

As we wait in the auditorium for the counselor, the movie screen on stage displays the Home Shopping Network.

Down the left side of the screen is an advertisement for "the Cure" for $29.99. It doesn't say what the cure is for, but I'm thinking sarcastically it's a hell of a lot cheaper than the one I'm getting.

Fred, the counselor, arrives and starts the session. He is medium height, stocky. Wears glasses, has a gravelly voice and a folksy way of talking.

One of his suggestions for relapse prevention is to make a HALT card. HALT stands for feeling Hungry, Angry, Lonely, Tired. These are the biggest causes of relapse. His advice is to determine in advance how you will handle any one of these things.

When you feel like taking a drink, you should break out the HALT card, try to figure out which symptom you are feeling at that moment, and take care of it:

Are you Hungry? Eat. Pack some snacks. Prepare some meals in advance. Don't skip meals.

Are you Angry? Try to determine in advance how you will handle your anger. Can you work or run it off, confront, count to 10, take deep breaths, listen to music, go to church?

Are you Lonely? Communicate with someone in any way: phone, visit, e-mail, join a chat room. Call someone's phone number even if you know they're not home, just to hear a voice. Talk to someone. Fred mentions that alcoholics are the only people who treat loneliness with isolation. Who you gonna call? Fred volunteers himself. Anytime.

Are you Tired? How can you get some rest right now? Not necessarily sleep, but how can you take a break and get reenergized? Deep breathing? Stretching? Plan for it.

Each of the factors of HALT will apply at one time or another. Thinking about how you'll handle these things in advance can help when the urge to drink arises.

This makes sense to me. One of my biggest triggers is

being tired. I've fought insomnia for years. I would go to bed at 10, still be awake at 3 a.m. It's often after one or two weeks of this, when I'm totally strung out and exhausted, that I head to a bottle to knock me out. I could write a book on the things I've done to try to get a good night's rest, but I've found some help recently by seeing a sleep specialist.

Being hungry is another story. I don't think my blood sugar's been normal in decades. I have to work really hard not to get hungry, to keep my blood sugar level stable, or I'm stopping for a bottle before I even realize it. I decide to make my diet my number-one priority when I get out.

One of my biggest triggers is really weird: it's being happy. Whenever I start to feel really good mentally or physically, I inevitably turn to the bottle. I just don't know how to handle the happiness thing. I don't know what to do with it.

Since that trigger is not included on Fred's HALT card example, I make my own and add an "ED" at the end: HALT(ED). The ED stands for ElateD. I need to work on figuring out what to do when I'm happy.

His next topic on relapse prevention is the "Consequence Card." The objective of the card is to stop you from taking that first drink by listing all the consequences that would occur if you did. If you still have the urge to drink even after reading your HALT (ED) card, you're supposed to read the "Consequences Card". What will happen to you as a result should be meaningful to your life, powerful enough to stop you from reaching for that drink. "My husband will be pissed at me" probably will not do it. "I will lose custody of my kids" just might. Here is the "Consequences Card" I made up while I sat there:

MY CONSEQUENCES CARD

> I will lose my sobriety.
> I will lose the respect of my husband, kids, and friends.
> I will disappoint my family and friends.
> I will lose control over myself.
> I will feel bad physically, mentally, emotionally, and spiritually.
> I will lose my job with the best company I've ever worked for.
> I will lose my life.
> I will die like my brothers.
> I won't live to see my grandchildren.
> When I die, I will break my kids' and husband's heart.
> When I die, my mother will give up and die too.

When the session ends, I continue to sit there staring at the page I've written, until dinner is announced. I walk slowly to the dining room, still thinking about my very real consequences.

I sit in the dining room at a table with other patients. We're called to the counter one at a time to pick up our plates: individual Cornish hens, roasted potatoes, peas and carrots, a flaky biscuit, tossed salad with ranch dressing, and vanilla ice cream with orange sherbet for dessert. It's good, really good!

Back in my room, I work more on my affirmations until the announcement is made: **"Tonight's movie, 'The Days of Wine and Roses', will be shown in the auditorium in 15 minutes. All patients,** except detox patients, **are invited to attend."**

Having never seen it, I head downstairs to the darkened auditorium. I'm the only one there! It feels weird but also good because I don't feel like talking right now.

The movie really hits home. It's in black and white, takes place in the '50s or '60s.

Young Jack Lemmon and Lee Remick play incredibly realistic alcoholics. I identify with their denial, portrayed so vividly in the scene where, after months of being sober, Joe (Jack Lemmon) sneaks two bottles of alcohol taped to the insides of his calves into the room he shares with Kiersten (Lee Remick) in her father's house.

He bought the booze in celebration of their being sober and hard working for months. They're going to reward themselves with just a "tiny bit" of booze.

The bottles are quickly gone; Joe and Kiersten are drunk out of their minds. But those two bottles are not enough, of course. They never are.

How many times have I bought some booze, thinking I'd have just a little bit—one drink—only to wake up having lost one, two, three days to drinking?

When the movie ends, I pass the crowded nurses' station. Apparently Friday night is a big night for checking in. There are several good-looking young men standing there. Some are well known to the nurses. I'm hoping they're here for recaps and not relapse.

I journal for a little while in my room. I'm thinking, this rehab stuff isn't so bad—I've had a pretty good day!

DAY TWO

6:15 a.m. Vital signs are taken. The aide reminds me to be up by seven and to drink at least 64 ounces of clear fluids before my Duffy treatment, time unknown. I can have jello and broth, brought to me on a tray. Before I leave my room, an aide comes in with a round blue plastic basin that she sets on the floor next to my bed atop a towel.

An ominous sign.

I grab a pink plastic pitcher and a straw like the ones I saw the other patients with yesterday. I fill it with PowerAde and ice.

This morning, the breakfast announcement is clearly not meant for me, so the only thing I have to do until treatment is to see a video called "Humor Your Stress".

Almost all of the patients show up, sign in. Many have pitchers like mine. We sit, sip, watch the video. It's just okay, not hilarious. In fact, by the time the video is over, the room is just about empty. I mean, how funny can anything be while you're waiting to throw up?

I feel bloated with PowerAde, and as I walk up the stairs, I can smell the strong odor of alcohol. Standing at the nurses' station, I can see into a room with bottles lined up on a counter. I'm getting nauseated already. I walk over to the room.

"Do you know when I'll be getting my treatment?" I ask the woman inside. It's after 10 a.m., and I'm anxious to see what it's all about, get on with it.

"Not too much longer," she replies. "I'm Diane, the treatment nurse, and I'll be doing your CCT (author's note: Counter Conditioning Treatment) today."

We shake hands.

I return to my room and think about my sons. They have no idea I'm here.

I call my oldest son, Mike, 27, to tell him. He gets angry.

"How come nobody told me how bad you are?"

I'm thinking: Because nobody wants to face it. And nobody knows what to do about it. And I think they are ashamed. We don't talk about it, just as we never talked about my father's problem when I was a kid. We'd acknowledge that Dad was drunk, and we'd steer clear of him, but that's as far as it went.

"Are you gonna get fired, Mom, for taking all this time off?"

I'm telling him I'm trying to fix my life, and he's asking about my job. Now I'm getting angry. "Mike, it's okay. I don't think that's going to happen, but it's a chance I have to take. My life is more important than my job."

Mike and I are very close. I understand his anger. He doesn't want his mom to be a drunk. He doesn't want me to be in this position. He hurts for me. He hurts for him.

I tell him about the program. He is very, very skeptical. "It doesn't sound like anything I've ever heard of. How did you find this place?"

I can't talk anymore. I believe in what I'm doing, but I can't defend it right now. "I have to go, Mike. I love you. Please call me once in a while."

"I love you too, Mom. And I will call."

That was rougher than I thought it would be, but I have to get this over with. I call my son Craig, 25. Craig has seen me drunk more often than Mike, less often than Carolyn. I explain the same thing to him—where I am, what I'm doing. Why.

"That's great, Mom," he exclaims. "You're getting the help you need!"

I'm so relieved at his reaction. I tell him I love him, hang up. Cry.

I need to get myself under control, change my mood. Now that I know what my treatment is about, I become a little obsessed with the term "throwing up". I'm thinking people here probably have some more creative words for it, so I decide to ask them for help creating a list of synonyms.

At 11:05 a.m., Diane comes to my room to lead me to treatment. It's a small room, maybe eight feet by eight feet. On my left is a chair set in front of a three-foot-wide counter with a stainless steel basin set into the center. A small round trash receptacle sits to the right of the chair. On the wall in front of me is a huge mirror. To the right is a taller counter containing all types of liquor bottles.

Diane is a pretty, petite, fifty-ish woman with blonde hair and a deceptively small voice.

"This is the emetic drug," she says, pouring a small amount of clear fluid into two 8-ounce glasses half-filled with water. "We add a pinch of salt to cut the bitterness."

She hands them to me. "Drink this down," she says.

The liquid is thick and bitter, despite the salt.

She tells me there's an eight-minute wait until the drug takes effect. She asks for my drink of choice and the brand of alcohol.

"Tanqueray Gin and tonic with a slice of lemon."

She wants to know if there is any other alcohol I like that I've drunk in the past four months.

"Vodka and tequila."

She gets the gin bottle, sets up four glasses: two 6-ounce sizes, two 8-ounce. She fills them halfway with water.

I want to know if I can have them mixed with tonic. She says no—they are not trying to make this a pleasurable experience!

"Why the different sized glasses?"

"We alternate sizes because we found it helps patients drink them down better."

Then she pours gin into each one. She tells me I will have to guzzle them.

I'm a little surprised at that and tell her so.

"Did you understand the treatment before you came here?" she asks kindly.

Well, I did, but until now I've avoided thinking about exactly what that means.

"Yes," I answer meekly.

"Tomorrow you'll have to drink more—we increase the amount at each treatment. We'll mix it up a little. You'll get mostly gin, tomorrow we'll add vodka, then wine and beer, then the tequila."

Before I have a chance to digest her words, she says: "Here we go: Drink up!"

I chug the first glass without stopping.

LET THE NAUSEA BEGIN

Halfway through the second glass, I have to stop to throw up. It's orange colored—the PowerAde—and it gets up my nose.

"Relax," she says.

Right.

"Get your breath, then guzzle. You have to drink quickly. We don't want the alcohol to get into your system."

She hands me a tissue to blow my nose. I look at my red face in the mirror—my eyes are tearing, my dirty-blond hair disheveled. My mouth has formed into a grimace.

I chug and throw up, throw up and chug, until all the glasses are empty.

The first part of treatment is over.

Diane walks me back to my room. She tells me I'll be sick on and off for three more hours; that it will come in waves."

She writes the time my treatment will end—2:30—on a piece of paper, tapes the paper on the nightstand where I can see it. She sets a gin-soaked rag next to the pillow, tells me part of my treatment is to breathe the fumes while I lie there so the discomfort level is increased.

"We want you to be nauseated the whole three hours."

Before closing the door, she adds, "Think about your addiction."

I'm so happy to have my watch on. I stare at it, willing the time to pass. "Three hours, three hours," I keep repeating to myself. "This will last only three hours. I can take it for three hours."

But time passes slowly.

I heave into the basin. I am sweating, my body shivering as the sweat dries.

So hot, so cold. Sick.

In between heaves, I think about my drinking habits.

I'm a "closet" binge drinker. I take great pains to hide my booze (as though anyone's really fooled). I spend a lot of time in our spare room, telling my family "I don't feel good" or "I'm so tired I need to be by myself." My excuses have gotten more elaborate, wild. I need to write them down so I can remember to whom I told what. Sometimes in the morning I can't even read my writing.

When I get into the spare room, I read and drink, drink and read, then just drink until I pass out. I burn a candle to hide the smell, hide my glass under the blankets in case someone comes in unexpectedly. How many times have I soaked myself with booze, spilling my glass in my hurry to hide it? I wonder why I've never burned myself with the candle.

I hide my bottles under the bed, except when I have to leave the room. Then they go under the pillows, where no one has yet found them. I learned to do that after my husband, Gary, confiscated my under-the-bed stash once too often. I'm perversely proud of the fact that I outsmart him.

Though he takes my liquor whenever he finds it, Gary never talks to me about my drinking except to ask, "Why, Kath? What made you take that first drink?"

As if any of this is rational. As if when I intellectually identify a "reason," I will stop. Can stop.

Nurses and aides stop in frequently to monitor my pulse and level of nausea on a scale of 0 to 3.

"2," I croak.

A little later: "How's your nausea now?"

"Still 2," I tell her.

As soon as she leaves the second time, I panic. Should I have told her 3? Will they do something more to me tomorrow to get me to a 3?

Time goes by slowly, s-l-o-w-l-y. I smell the gin from the rag and from the basin. And throw up some more.

I report my nausea levels: 1.5, 1.5, 0.5.

A nurse comes in at 2:30 to tell me my treatment is over. I fall asleep, wake up at 3:45, think about the treatment.

Surreal.

Incredibly, I feel fine when I get up. I hurry to the dining room to get something to eat before the next mandatory class at 4:30.

COUNSELOR'S CHOICE LECTURE

The mandatory lecture "Counselor's Choice" is held in the recreation room outside the auditorium. People are seated around the ping-pong table and in chairs lined up against the walls.

Judy, a pretty, slightly plump counselor with long, silky blonde hair and a kind, gentle manner, has chosen to talk about relapse prevention as Fred did yesterday. But instead of giving a lecture, she asks us what we think will work for us to prevent relapse.

She wants participation. No one's giving her any.

"So," she says, "since you seem shy with each other, we're going to play a game to get to know one another. Let's arrange the chairs in a big circle away from the table."

The groaning and eye rolling start.

She explains the game. There will be one less chair than there are patients. The patient without the chair will stand in the middle of the circle and ask a question of the group. Everyone who can answer a "yes" to the question has to get up and find a new seat. The person left standing asks the next question.

It would be hard to find a less enthusiastic group than this mixed-gender, institutional-pajamas-and-robe-clad collection of addicts who have either been throwing up, receiving Faradic treatment, or sleeping off sedation therapy.

But we have no choice—we have to play. A young man volunteers to ask the first question: "Who is a multi-substance user?"

People quickly shuffle around. One is left standing.

"Who has ever gotten up not knowing where they were?"

Shuffle, shuffle.

One poor guy—he can't be more than 21—seems to be moving to every question; others move only occasionally.

I have to get up only once: "Who has been drunk before breakfast?" And I lose my seat.

As corny as it is, the game really does break the ice. We laugh a lot at ourselves, good-naturedly at each other.

Dinnertime: shrimp fettuccini with bread sticks and tossed salad. After the day I had, the thick white sauce is not at all appetizing. I think to myself, they need to take this off the menu completely! I eat only the shrimp and salad, drink a cup of tea.

I sit with some other new patients and we talk about our day, trying not to get too graphic.

I leave dinner with Mary, who's in the room next to mine. Mary is a frail woman with short, brown, pixie hair. Wrinkled face, sallow skin. Her eyes have huge dark shadows underneath. She's been here five days detoxing. Today she had her first Duffy, but she is in such bad physical shape she doesn't have to swallow any alcohol. She only has to swish and spit. This is her first trip downstairs, and she is feeling particularly vulnerable.

I help her find her room, tell her to call me if she needs anything. I return to my own room for my journal, and head out to the deck.

Outside I talk with Chet, whose room is kitty-corner to mine. We have bonded playing musical chairs. He was admitted at the same time as I was, which means our schedules are identical.

Chet is a big, handsome man with wavy, prematurely gray hair, maybe early 40s. He talks to me a little about his kids, how he's missing his daughter moving into her freshman college dorm this weekend. He's here instead. He's feeling bad about that, but I congratulate him. Tell him I think it'll mean more to her in the long run.

We compare treatment notes. He had a really bad time—he was sick for the whole three hours and then some. Shyly, he asks if I got diarrhea from the treatment the way he did.

"No," I answer, "just the nausea."

When it gets dark, we return to our rooms. On the way, I check tomorrow's schedule at the nurses' station. My Duffy is listed for the afternoon. The nurse tells me I can have breakfast at 7 a.m.

I'm thrilled to be able to eat, but also annoyed because I like to get things over with so I can relax.

I call Gary and my friend Lynn to check in. Watch television for a while, take my meds, go to sleep. I'm exhausted.

DAY THREE

At 6:45 a.m., my vital signs are taken. Still good. I have to ask the nurse what date it is—I'm losing track already.

In the bathroom, I look at myself in the mirror. My brown eyes are puffy, slightly bloodshot; my face is red. My ears still hurt from throwing up yesterday.

After hearing the breakfast announcement, I head down to the dining room for some French toast, bacon, tea. I sit with Sam and Robert, both of whom I got to know after the musical chairs game.

Sam, a tall, slightly stocky 20-something with dark buzz-cut hair, is an artist. I think how neat it would be if I did decide to publish my journal if another patient would illustrate it. I mention it. He's not at all interested.

Robert is medium height, medium build, in his 60s with white hair, a healthy complexion, glasses. He has an air of professionalism about him. He talks a little about his alcohol addiction. This is his second stint at Schick Shadel. After his first treatment, he was sober for 14 years, after which time he thought he had conquered his problem and took just one drink. Eight years and many, many drinks later, he's back at Schick Shadel.

After breakfast I hit the area where the water pitchers are kept. Several patients are standing around. I tell them I didn't like my experience with the PowerAde yesterday.

"Don't drink that stuff. The best thing is to drink gallons

and gallons of water. Drink even more than they say," one guy advises me. "It'll really help ease the discomfort."

This advice sounds pretty good, so I grab a pitcher, fill it with water, and leave, feeling like I'm getting to know the ropes.

The morning's video is "Cross Addiction".

The doctor in the film tells us that if you give up your addictive substance(s) and start using another, before long you will either be back to using your old substance again or addicted to the new one.

A substance by any other name…

I have smoked marijuana only a few times in my life, the last time decades ago. But before I came to treatment, I thought my "safety net" was that if I gave up booze, I could smoke pot sometimes when I really need to relax. Or get high. I really thought it would be possible.

It isn't.

For the first time in my life, I am realizing how powerful and real my addiction is. That I am addicted.

I am addicted to alcohol! I've said it before, but I'm just now realizing what it means. I cannot sample, taste, try, use anything. Ever.

Halfway through the video, I have to get up to use the bathroom. I see a man seated in the back row, aisle seat, with a walker next to him. He has long, gray-streaked dark hair that he wears pulled back into a ponytail. His strong facial features suggest he is Native American. He smiles shyly at me as I walk by.

"Can I bring you back a glass of water?" How difficult it must be for him to manage his water and his walker.

His gratitude at this simple gesture is almost

42

embarrassing, and I am humbled, reminded that it is the simple things we do that are the most meaningful.

After the video I'm back in my room for only a few minutes when Gary, who introduces himself as my counselor, walks in. I think about his name—how it's not all that common—yet in my life my husband, my deceased brother, and now my counselor share it.

"After reading your history, I thought you would get a lot out of this book," he says.

I'm so impressed. Expecting to see a book on PTSD, child abuse, or alcoholism, I glance at the cover: "Mutant Message from Down Under".

"What? What the hell is this?" I'm thinking to myself.

But I smile and politely ask out loud: "How does this relate to me?"

"Take from it whatever you want" is his cryptic response.

Our session lasts for about two and a half hours. Several times I have to leave to refill my water pitcher in preparation for my afternoon Duffy. Or to relieve myself in the hall bathroom of some of the fluid I've already drunk.

Gary is a good-looking man in his 40s, sandy-brown hair, a small port-wine stain on his left cheek. He speaks in a kind of slurry drawl, though I can't place the accent.

He asks me questions I've been asked before and then some. As we talk, he begins suggesting things for me to do once I leave: get a personal trainer to advise me how to eat while working out, read some books he recommends, attend Monday-evening meetings at Schick Shadel, address my marital discord and PTSD with a therapist.

As he talks, my mind wanders ahead to this afternoon when I'll be doing my Duffy. It's on the quantity of fluids I'm supposed to be drinking. I'm wondering if I'll be properly prepared, and I'm a little anxious.

"You are a story of your own creation," he continues. "If you don't like the story you have, rewrite it."

"Huh?" My attention once again focuses on him. "Can you give me an example?"

"So your father was an alcoholic and he abused you. That's your story, the one I read in your history. If you don't like it, make up a new one. Like: 'My father had a disease. He loved me, but he couldn't always show it. He couldn't get the help he needed to become the father I wanted.' That's your new story. You are whatever story you write."

He gives me homework if I want to do it—to rewrite my story, work on deconstructing some of my automatic responses to stress and disappointments.

He draws a lot of pictures. Shows me how, at the center, we are all spiritual human beings. As we talk, he gets excited for me. "You are really into this. You are really going to enjoy your recovery, I can tell."

"You are perfect!" he says, leaving.

Wow! First, I have great veins. Then Ruby tells me it's all about me. And now Gary tells me I'm perfect! This place is good for my ego.

I start right in on the exercises Gary gave me. Diane stops by to tell me she is getting ready for me now.

Is "Thanks" the appropriate response?

She comes back a few minutes later, leads me to the same treatment room as yesterday. I sit down and remove my glasses—ready as I'll ever be.

"Drink Up!" she says, handing the first glass of medicine to me.

I guzzle two half-glasses of water with the emetic and

salt. While we wait the eight minutes for the drug to take effect, she again sets up the bar for my session.

Diane is a very sweet woman doing an incredibly bizarre job. My sense of humor ignites briefly as I wonder how she describes it to people. A vision of her being interviewed by David Letterman passes through my mind: "Let me get this straight," Dave says. "You give alcohol to drunks and then watch them throw up? How great is that?" he asks with his goofy grin.

To do this job day after day, with such caring and professionalism, she must have a strong sense of perspective, knowing how much she helps people in the long run. And she must have a great sense of humor!

My own humor vanishes as quickly as it came as I'm snapped back to the business at hand. I'm not very talkative, an unusual state for me. And though I'm trying hard not to be hostile, I'm not very friendly.

"I'm actually a very nice person," I say apologetically. "I know you can't tell by my behavior."

"Don't worry about it," she responds. "Everybody acts differently in here. This is a very emotional room. Lots of stuff comes up."

I can interpret that statement in sooooo many ways!

It's time to start drinking. Today I'll have gin, vodka, end with gin.

She hands me the first glass.

"Drink up," she says.

I guzzle.

Second glass—I guzzle.

I pause to take a breath.

Third glass—chug!

"Yesterday you brought it up really quickly, which is good

because we don't want that alcohol staying around. If you don't bring something up soon, I'll have to ask you to induce vomiting."

By that she means stick a tongue depressor down my throat.

I drink the fourth glass. Halfway through, I nearly knock my chair over exploding to my feet by the force of my heaving!

I continue to retch. My stomach is sore. My breath comes in gasps. I see a contorted face in the mirror—red, swollen.

My throat is sore. Fluid goes up my nose. I cough.

Five and a half glasses down. I'm panting. For a few minutes I hold the glass to my lips, unable to drink one more drop; Diane tells me if I can't swallow any more to smell, swish, and spit the alcohol into the basin. I gratefully, almost enthusiastically, follow her instructions before she has a chance to change her mind.

I continue to retch, bringing up huge quantities of fluid. When a spasm subsides, she walks me back to my room, tapes the little sign on the nightstand indicating my treatment will be over at 4:40 p.m.

My room has been set up as yesterday: basin on the floor sitting on a towel. She places the gin-soaked rag next to my head, prepares to leave.

"Someone will come by in a half hour to give you a butterfly."

"What's a butterfly?" I whisper hoarsely.

"It's beer mixed with more of the emetic drug. Because you've ingested more alcohol, we need to be sure you get it all up.

"Why is it called a butterfly?" My voice is barely audible, but I'm curious.

"We call it a butterfly because of the way it makes your stomach flutter after drinking it.

Oh.

I throw up twice before my nurse, Brandon, comes in with the butterfly.

"Sit up," he commands, not unkindly. "I need you to drink this in one gulp. Bottoms up!"

I drink it down.

It is so gross.

Today is different from yesterday. I don't throw up much, even after the butterfly. But I'm still nauseated and there's a gurgling in my intestines. I think I'll soon be experiencing the diarrhea Chet talked about yesterday.

Sure enough, the need becomes urgent.

I barely make it to the bathroom.

When I'm done, I stumble back to bed.

A short time later, another nurse comes in to check my pulse, my nausea level.

"It's a 1. But I do have diarrhea," I add.

I continue to purge from both ends until empty at last, I ring the nurse's bell to ask for clean pajamas and a robe.

Brandon quickly returns with them.

I still have 20 minutes to go before the treatment ends, so I wash up, change my clothes, and sit in the chair, waiting.

Once released I shower, come back to my now immaculately sanitized room, and sleep for a few minutes until dinner.

Once again, I can't believe I have no residual nausea. And I can't believe how hungry I am!

But I can only get down a few bites.

I nap some more after dinner. Wake at 7 p.m. feeling a lot better. Help myself to some sandwiches from the food cart that appears nightly as if by magic—loaded with all sorts of good food for people who have missed meals throughout the day.

My husband and daughter come around 7:30 p.m. Gary is going away on a business trip for the whole week, so this is my only opportunity to see him.

He brought me the socks I asked for, as well as the Sunday New York Times crossword puzzle, which I work faithfully every week. I am touched he remembered to bring it.

I wasn't expecting Carolyn, and I'm delighted to see her.

We talk a little about the past two days. I see Carolyn turning a little green at my graphic descriptions, but they seemed interested (and sometimes amused) nonetheless.

I tell them I'm collecting synonyms for throw up. Gary and Carolyn add "york," "barf," and "yak" to my list. I ask Carolyn to come back at 8 a.m. tomorrow for Dr. Smith's lecture: "Medical Aspects of Addiction and Treatment." I need my family to understand my problem, and she's the only one available. She eagerly agrees, anxious to learn more about me.

And herself.

They leave at 9 p.m. when visiting hours are over.

I read the book "Mutant Message from Down Under"— trying to figure out how it relates to me—until I fall asleep.

DAY FOUR

6:30 a.m. My vital signs are taken: temperature 97.6 degrees, blood pressure (B/P) 122/69, pulse 75. A nurse gives me my morning meds. I weigh 159.

Since I am having my sedation interview today, I can't eat or drink anything—not even water—but I'm not complaining. Today has to be an easier day than the past two!

At 7:45 a.m. Carolyn arrives for the lecture, and we head down to the auditorium.

Dr. Smith is the Chief of Staff of Schick Shadel. He's been here for 45 years, has published many articles on alcoholism. He is a kindly, soft-spoken man with gray hair, "cheaters" on the end of his nose. Behind the glasses are gentle blue eyes. He begins:

Roughly one person out of every ten drinkers in the United States is an alcoholic. There are 3.3 million problem drinkers among youth in the 14- to 17-year-old age range. These drinkers become alcoholics regardless of their IQ or education level.

People in lower income brackets have a lower-than-average rate of alcoholism, while those in the higher-income brackets have a higher-than-average rate. This may be because they have more money to spend or tend to be in social settings where drinking is routine.

In the United States, the highest rates of alcoholism occur in the Eskimo or Native American populations. Of the Caucasians, people with Celtic ancestors (Irish, Scottish) have the highest rates. Scandinavian, American blacks, and Hispanic Americans also have high rates.

I think about this. I am fully half-Irish, my father having immigrated to this country in his teens.

Dr. Smith continues:

The incidence of alcoholism or predisposition to alcoholism is less prevalent in those with English or Middle European ancestry. Italian Americans are well below average. Those of Asian descent are even lower. The lowest levels are people of Orthodox Jewish descent. The figures for the United States are reflected in the worldwide statistics on alcoholism.

Various explanations have been offered for this: the type of alcohol ("hard liquor" versus beer or wine), cultural or religious customs, the age at which drinking was introduced. Most of these theories have long been disproved.

Higher or lower incidences of other diseases—diabetes, some types of anemia, Buerger's disease (acute inflammation and clotting of arteries and veins affecting the hands and feet), to name a few—also occur in different ethic groups, so alcoholism is not unique in showing differences in susceptibility among different population groups. The population with the lowest incidence of alcoholism originated in those parts of the world where alcohol has been available in relatively large quantities for the greatest number of generations.

The Mediterranean region has had alcohol for about 15,000 years, according to archaeological evidence. On the other hand, large amounts of alcohol became available to northern Europeans (e.g., Scandinavians) only about 1,200-1,500 years ago.

Eskimo and Native American populations have had ready access to alcohol only since the European colonization of the North American continent. For some Native American populations, this exposure has been only in the past 300-400 years, whereas Eskimos have been exposed for less than 100 years.

This appears to demonstrate the evolutionary process of "natural selection." The Mediterranean populations most susceptible to alcoholism probably died out over the many generations during which alcohol was consumed. North American Indians have had very few generations during which to develop an alcoholism-resistant racial strain.

Dr. Smith's comments bring back memories of a visit I took to explore my roots when I was a teenager. I stayed with my Aunt Winnie on a farm outside a small town in Northern Ireland. Evenings we went to the nearby inn, a place where the Irish locals sang raucously while others played the concertina and most everyone lifted their pints.

I was introduced to the innkeeper's son, Sean, who told me he had taken the pledge, part of an Irish abstinence movement founded in the late 1800s by Father Cullen, a member of the Society of Jesus. Father Cullen recognized the dangers of alcohol—so much harm had been caused by the drunkenness so prevalent in Ireland at the time. At first he appealed for total abstinence just to people who abused alcohol, but later he appealed to everyone to abstain in an effort to support those with problems. And to prevent others from developing problems.

At that time, Sean had never had any alcohol and, from his experience as the innkeeper's son watching alcohol's effects on the patrons, had pledged never to touch a drop.

Several decades later, I learned from my aunt that Sean was a hopeless alcoholic...

Carolyn is paying strict attention to the lecture. As I learn more about alcoholism, I am so happy to have her by my side.

She asks Dr. Smith a question about gender. He tells her that male alcoholics usually outnumber females by a ratio of 5 to 1, though that's not true of the audience this morning.

I can see she's concerned for herself. For her brothers.

When the lecture is over, we talk a little bit about what we learned.

Carolyn leaves and I head back to my room to read my affirmations before my sedation interview. We were asked to select from a list of affirmations provided and told we could add our own, for a total of 24.

Here is a sampling of the affirmations we could choose from:

1. I choose not to have my disease control or manipulate me.
2. I am a success in all that I do.
3. I enjoy my life without alcohol or other drugs.
4. I enjoy being alive.
5. I balance my life with work and play.
6. I enjoy a steady flow of positive energy.
7. I am loved, accepted, acknowledged, and appreciated.
8. I am clever and creative; I am engaged by life.
9. I have an awesome connection with my higher power.
10. I love, forgive and accept my self unconditionally.
11. My inner vision is always clear and focused.
12. Today I choose new responses to old situations.
13. I am a spiritual being.
14. I'm comfortable in every situation without alcohol or drugs.
15. I now attract caring and supportive relationships into my life.

16. Alcohol and drugs are repulsive to me.
17. I don't allow other people, places, things or thoughts to have power over me.

There are also spaces on the form where you can write in your own. I want mine to be very specific so I write them on a separate piece of paper:

MY AFFIRMATIONS

1. I love being sober!
2. I enjoy my sobriety more each day.
3. I am a worthy, capable and valuable person.
4. I enjoy my life without alcohol or drugs.
5. I calmly accept the things I cannot change.
6. I respond peacefully to any and all stressful situations in life.
7. I fall asleep quickly and rest comfortably through the night.
8. I wake up every day refreshed and filled with enthusiasm.
9. I enjoy relationships with other people.
10. Every day I appreciate and celebrate my sobriety.
11. I am thrilled to be alive and well!
12. I enjoy a steady flow of positive energy.
13. I love, forgive, and accept myself unconditionally.
14. I am at peace with my past and forgiving of those in my past.
15. I create exciting purpose and meaning in my life.
16. My inner vision is always clear and focused.
17. I make the right life choices for me without using alcohol.

18. I love to eat and drink only healthy foods in moderation.
19. My weight and muscle mass are stable and right where they should be for me.
20. I eat slowly, chewing every bite.
21. I have a multitude of positive life interests and relationships.
22. I radiate success, confidence, and enthusiasm.
23. My self-talk is always positive.
24. I am lovable, loving, and loved.

In the treatment room, I sit in a comfortable reclining chair. The nurse starts an IV, while the counselor (Judy of the "Musical Chairs" game) sits at a computer ready to key in my responses to the questions they'll ask. I hand her my list of affirmations to review.

You are allowed to submit your own questions in addition to the affirmations. Which I did. I'm interested to know what my subconscious "thinks" about my marriage and my career.

Judy is pleased that I have submitted my own questions as well as a personalized list of affirmations. Once the IV is in and the medication is running into my arm, she gives me back the list and asks me to read them aloud.

I get to about number six. The next thing I know, I'm being wheeled back to my room. I remember nothing. Not one thing! This is normal, since Versed is an amnesiac drug. But it's very weird. I ask Judy what I said, but she said they'll review the results with me tomorrow, since experience has shown I won't remember what she tells me if she tells me too soon after treatment.

For the sake of clarity, I include the results here rather than in the actual chronological sequence they were given to me.

The first question is this: "On a scale of 1 to 10, 1 being weak and 10 being strong, what is your current level of aversion to alcohol or to drugs you are being treated for?"

My answer: 2!

I have thrown my guts up over the past two days, and I've only reached 2!

Other questions have to do with self-esteem (I said 6 on a scale of 1 to 10) and whether you had a happy childhood (I said no).

One of the questions I asked them to ask me was this: "Are you happy with your current occupation?"

I've thought about this so much lately. I work as a systems analyst for a great company. My employers like and respect me, give me all sorts of opportunities. And I have fabulous benefits. But I've been doing the same thing for 23 years. I've been using the left side of my brain so much, I'm afraid the right side has atrophied.

I see myself going to work another six years, when the house and Carolyn's college will be paid off, when I can "retire" from my present job. This vision makes me despair because I have a lot of creative ideas and energy that I think might be better spent working more with people.

All these thoughts come tumbling out during my interview. I'm not surprised by my response. But I still don't know what to do about it.

I was surprised by my answer to only one question: "How long has your chemical use been a problem for you?"

My response was: "Probably since I was 16."

If you had asked me that question while I was not under the effects of the drug, I might have said, "The past 10 years since my brothers died." But thinking about it now, I realize I never drank "normally." From the first moment I took a drink—before age 12 at Christmas at my house, allowed to have a whiskey and ginger ale to celebrate the holiday—I drank to excess.

I remember a New Year's Eve at Bear Mountain Inn in New York when I was 17, lying under the dining table so drunk I was unable to move. So badly hung over I couldn't get out of bed for two days. I start remembering other dates, other dinners, lunches! Other parties.

I begin to remember warnings from friends about the frequency and quantity of my drinking. Warnings I so easily dismissed.

I recall countless phone calls I made the morning after, checking in with friends to make sure I had done nothing the night before to jeopardize our friendship. Or to make a fool of myself.

The evidence of the length and severity of my addiction just keeps piling up…

Dr. Smith makes his rounds and shares the results of my blood work with me.

He has great news: all my blood work, with two exceptions, is normal. I was concerned about my liver, but aside from being enlarged, it is showing no signs of damage.

One of the abnormal tests is a direct result of alcohol consumption: triglycerides. Upper normal range for this test is 150. Mine is high, at 200 milligrams per deciliter. High triglycerides are risk factors in heart disease and strokes. Dr. Smith assures me that the triglycerides will return to normal once I stop drinking.

The other abnormal result is cholesterol. Normal is under 200. Greater than 239 is considered high. Mine is 273.

High cholesterol runs in my family. Dr. Smith tells me diet can correct only half the problem; the rest is due to genetics, and he strongly urges me to discuss this with my family doctor once I'm released.

YOU ARE WHAT YOU EAT (AND DRINK)

At 4:15 we sign in for a mandatory nutrition lecture.

I've always felt nutrition and food chemistry play a far greater part in our health than is acknowledged. When I gave up smoking and started gaining weight at age 21, I decided I needed to learn something about nutrition. I never dreamed I would put it to use keeping myself alive and not using it to live my healthiest life possible.

I believe if I hadn't known as much as I do about food and its effects on and in the body, I'd be in a lot worse shape by now. I know drinking dehydrates you, so I drink lots of water to rehydrate myself. I know alcohol washes vitamins out of the body, so I take extra B vitamins and folic acid. When I'm sober, I eat really well: healthy, lean cuts of meat, chicken, salads, fruits.

My father suffered a seizure once while withdrawing from alcohol. I was the only one home at the time—I couldn't have been more than about 10. I called 911, cried hysterically in the ambulance and at the hospital. He recovered with no permanent damage (at least, none that wasn't there before the seizure), but I've never forgotten that day, living in fear that one day it will happen to me when I'm withdrawing from a binge. So I take calcium-magnesium supplements because I read somewhere they can help prevent alcohol withdrawal seizures.

Even so, whenever I drink, especially recently, when my binges have been more frequent, longer lasting, and more ferocious, I'm scared.

So my interest in the topic of nutrition makes me pay strict attention. I'm the choir—preach to me!

The dietician tells us that alcohol affects nearly every part of our bodies, from digestion through losing brain cells. She gives us the U.S. Department of Agriculture food pyramid diagram along with the usual advice to eat lean meat, leafy green vegetables, more whole grains.

I ask her for some recipes or some specific suggestions about what to eat. I've heard the advice before. But how do you incorporate it into your life? What is a whole grain, anyway? What kind of green leafy vegetables?

Another thing I learn is that a diet of higher complex carbohydrates, moderate protein, and moderate fat seems to work best for the recovering alcoholic.

Because I am overweight by about 15 pounds and can't seem to lose them no matter what I do (I notice how giving up booze has not been a weight-loss option for me), I have been trying to avoid all other carbohydrates in my life. Or at least ones other than salad vegetables. But I crave them. During my sober cycles, if I exercise and don't eat carbs, something always feels missing. In fact, many times after exercising hard for several days in a row, then eating proteins and salads, my alcohol trigger goes off and I buy a bottle. My body is not satisfied—it craves sugar!

I sit and listen and feel my interest in nutrition rekindled. And a surprising thought pops into my head: I'd like to be up there giving this talk!

And I think: I bet I could do a good job.

The significance of this thought is profound. Is this the beginning of a goal, a dream? Am I actually seeing myself doing something besides drowning in alcohol?

As she nears the end of her lecture, dinner is announced. The group moves quickly, en masse, to the dining room. I'm not the only one who loves to eat.

The food is great: cole slaw, orange-flavored teriyaki chicken breast, rice, biscuits, and a small dessert of mandarin oranges in a creamy coconut sauce.

After dinner, I go out to the deck to write in my journal, half listening to others' stories, but not really participating.

At 7 p.m., an announcement is made: **"The graduates' and patients' meeting will begin in 15 minutes in the auditorium. All patients,** except detox patients, **are required to attend."**

This is one of three weekly support meetings held at Schick Shadel, and I'm anxious to see what it's all about.

As I settle into an inconspicuous chair, I watch the "townies" come in: former patients or neighborhood recovering/retired alcoholics/addicts. They are smiling, talking animatedly. The male inpatients walk in more slowly, talk less. The women inpatients enter in groups of twos and threes, chatting, seeming to gather strength and humor from each other.

I see the women making friends, bonding, and I feel a familiar sense of aloneness. Another familiar feeling—that of not being good enough—crops up and settles into place in the center of my rib cage.

I've never had many friends. I tell myself it's because I'm so independent that I've never needed or wanted many. But deep down I know the real reasons.

Growing up, I learned not to count on anyone but myself. My silent motto was: Don't ask for anything, and you won't be disappointed.

I remember an early incident with my mother that I think contributed significantly to my feelings.

I don't know how old I was—maybe eight or nine. My girlfriend Gloria who lived next door got a bike for Christmas. It was beautiful: teal blue, so shiny. And it had a horn—one of those round black plastic things you squeeze and it makes a honking noise like a goose.

Gloria would be out in the street with her father, who was teaching her how to ride. I wanted a bike too, so bad. I remember thinking that being able to get on something and ride wherever I wanted to—like around the block—would be the most wonderful thing in the world!

So I went home and asked for one. Probably begged; I don't remember. And one day my mother gave in and told me she would get one for me.

Another day she told me, "I ordered your bike. It should be delivered in a couple of weeks."

I was so happy—I just couldn't wait, even though I would've liked to have picked out the color myself.

But the bike didn't come.

And at least once a week I'd ask my mother about it.

"It took longer than they thought to get it in," she told me once.

Another time: "It broke coming off the truck. They had to order a new one."

Then she told me it was delivered to the wrong house.

I was recounting this latest problem to Gloria and her mother. Mrs. J. asked me where it was bought.

"Hin and Dickson," I told her.

She looked at me funny. "Hin and Dickson? That's a furniture store. They don't sell bikes there."

Confused, I ran home. My mother hemmed and hawed, but finally told me that there was no bike.

"But why did you tell me there was?"

I don't remember exactly what she said. What I do remember is the pain on her face, her eyes avoiding mine. Though I couldn't have put it into words at that age, I got it. I got that my mother was unable to face the fact that she couldn't get me something I wanted so badly, that she couldn't provide. And I learned it hurt my mother when I had wants, so from then on I tried not to have any. At least, none that she could see.

And I also developed trust issues.

The other reason I'm so "independent" is the shame that became ingrained. Growing up I was afraid to have kids over—they would see my drunken father, my dirty house, the four rooms that housed six people, the hide-a-bed left open, unmade in the living room. The bunk bed where I slept, sharing a room with a brother. No place to go, no place to play, no place to hide.

Except within.

So I've been scared. Terrified. That if people got to know me, they would discover the truth about me—that I'm not good enough, that I'm really a big phony, a piece of shit.

Scared too that if I got to know them, if I counted on them, they would let me down.

So I reject them before they can reject me, priding myself on my independence.

And tell myself it's okay.

At 7:15 p.m. sharp the meeting begins. Don is the substitute leader for this evening. He's a biker wearing black jeans, black T-shirt, black leather wristband with metal knobs. Black leather gloves with the fingers cut out. He has dark, curly hair that comes down to just past his chin. The only item of color is a red bandanna hanging out of his back pocket.

He opens the meeting with a few brief sentences: "Great to be sober. Getting better daily."

I notice he's fiddling with something.

"Let's make this a good meeting! Who wants to start?"

A hand goes up. Don flings the thing he's holding at the person. It's a rubber chicken. In order to talk, you have to be holding it.

People introduce themselves by their names and whatever else they want the group to know. No one says, "I'm Kathy and I'm an alcoholic," present tense. Some say they are retired, some are recovering, but no one *is*.

I like this. One of the problems I have with AA is having to say, "I am an alcoholic," because I believe in self-talk. What you tell yourself becomes the truth for you. I believe you are what you think you are, what you tell yourself you are.

I gave up smoking years ago. When talking about smoking, I don't say, "I am a smoker." Or "I am a recovering smoker." I say, "I used to smoke and I gave it up." That's where I want to be with alcohol. "I used to have a drinking problem and now I don't."

Am I kidding myself? I don't think so. I know now I can never have one drink, not one sip, just as I cannot take a drag from a cigarette, although I gave up smoking more than 35 years ago. But I don't want my life to be defined every waking moment by what was. I want to move on.

People tell their stories, share with us. The townies have lots of advice to offer those of us "still in pajamas." I listen with respect. The chicken gets hurled. Somewhere along the line, instead of tossing the chicken, someone merely hands it to the person next to him. And so on.

When my turn comes, I say: "My name is Kathy and I'm retiring my alcoholism this week."

A few claps, a few cheers.

"I came to this program because it seemed practical to

me. I'm working hard, doing all the things I've been told. I have a to do-list for when I get out. I've been doing the exercises and reading my packet."

Before I pass the chicken, I ask the group's help with my growing list of throw-up synonyms. Contributions include "spew" and "zook."

Someone volunteers "Buick," and I pass the chicken to the next person.

"Buick?"

There's lots of laughing at the meeting. Cross talk is allowed—if someone's having a problem, someone else might offer advice or things that worked for them.

I like this meeting. I resolve to attend once I'm a graduate.

After it ended, I get a snack, return to my room, write in my journal. Today was a great day—no Duffy.

I feel human.

DAY FIVE

The ringing of my cell phone awakens me in the dark. Where the hell is the damn thing? It's across the room, recharging. I stumble out of bed. "Hello?"

"Hi, Kath, it's me" comes the voice of my husband.

"What time is it?" I croak.

"It's 5:15. Listen, I'm in a hotel room in Idaho and I called the wrong number. I meant to call the guy I'm supposed to meet. Go back to sleep. I'm sorry."

But I can't get back to sleep. Today's another Duffy. I sit in my room, the hospital around me still nighttime quiet, and write.

Vitals are taken at 7: temp 97.6. I forget what my blood pressure is. Pulse 75. I weigh myself—158! I came in on Thursday at 165 and now weigh 158.

My Duffy breakfast tray is delivered to me: hot water with a packet of bouillon, plus jello. Although it's gold in color, I can't tell what flavor it is by eating it. I mix the bouillon and drink it. It's disgusting. Low sodium—what's the point?

When the morning's announcement about Dr. Smith's lecture is made, I put on my robe, fill a pitcher with water, head down to the auditorium. I notice the same thing as yesterday: the women are sitting in groups of twos and threes; the men sit with at least one space between them and the next person, perhaps only one or two per row. I sit in my usual place in the next to the last row—but I leave the aisle seat open for Carolyn.

64

Soft-spoken Dr. Smith begins the day's lecture on "Genetics and Addiction". I'm afraid for my children for what I know I'm going to hear. What I already know. What all of us here already know.

Carolyn slips in beside me shortly after he starts.

That alcoholism runs in families has been known since ancient times. A child born into a family with an alcoholic parent has a much greater chance of becoming an alcoholic than one born into a family with none. When either male or female alcoholics are studied, the rate of alcoholism in their close blood relatives is at least five times higher than would be expected in the general population.

That's certainly true in my family. Of my parents' four children, only my oldest brother, Terry, was spared. He seems to be able to take a drink or two. Or leave it.

Nature... or nurture?

Dr. Smith cites well-known studies to support the nature argument. Adoption studies comparing children whose biological parents included at least one known alcoholic with adoptees from nonalcoholic biological parents showed that the adoptees born of alcoholic parents had an alcoholism rate four times higher than that of children born of nonalcoholic parents.

Further adoption studies showed that even if children of at least one alcoholic parent were separated—one raised by their biological parents, and one adopted into a nonalcoholic family—there is no difference in the alcoholism rate between the two sets of siblings.

The best thing to do if you're an alcoholic, he says, is to keep your kids away from alcohol.

Patients shake their heads in frustration and sadness at the near impossibility of this.

"Talk to your kids all the time," he urges. "Don't be silent.

Warn them of the dangers. You have to try. Use yourselves as an example—the data is not in your favor."

The data is indeed stark. I worry about my oldest son, Mike. In college, he drank so much he gained about 15 pounds, his face bloated, his personality tensed. Since graduating, his drinking seems to have slowed down a lot. He is happy, healthy, physically fit, and in control. He can drink one or two drinks. He can also drink one or two six-packs.

I worry about my 25-year-old son, Craig, who seems to need a drink in his hand before he can be sociable.

I haven't worried too much about Carolyn because she had a lot of health problems in her teenage years that left her with a great appreciation for her health. She won't wreck it with alcohol.

I don't think.

I learn there are two types of alcoholics. Type 2 is handed down through the males of the family. It usually shows up before the age of 25, most frequently in the teen years. Males who develop this type of alcoholism are risk takers, usually have a few arrests early on.

A child of either sex can get Type 1. It generally shows up after the age of 25. For this type of alcoholism to manifest itself, a person needs to have both the genetic link and environmental stress.

I am obviously Type 1. My childhood was one big stress, and I have genetic links on both my father's and mother's sides through the males for as far back as anyone can remember.

I may be the first female in my family to be passing down this trait. I think my Irish Aunt Winnie drank a lot, but she didn't have kids. I'm the first female to graduate college and the first female I know of to pass on the alcoholic gene.

I feel tremendous guilt about this, although there's nothing I can do about it. But I see my kids' childhood faces in my mind, knowing that as adults they may have to struggle with this legacy as I am struggling now. I can't put into words how this feels.

I think about my mother, who lost two sons to addiction in the same year. My brother Mike was a year and a half older than me.

I've read that everyone fills a specific role in a family. Mike was my father's scapegoat. My father could go from zero to a red, raging, 60-mile-an-hour anger in just a few seconds when he had more than a few. And he always had more than a few. If Mike was around, he would get blamed for something. Anything. Didn't matter.

And then my father's belt would come off.

"Take your clothes off, boy," he'd say softly, ominously, the whites of his eyes growing larger.

While the rest of us watched, or hid, or cried, he would beat Mike's naked body with his leather belt. Once my mother got between them and the next thing I knew, she was on the floor.

Mike's tearful, hurt face and body jerking convulsively with every slap of the belt have haunted me all my life. I got hit with the belt too, but nothing like what Mike got.

So he was the one who always got into trouble—challenging, pushing the envelope. He seemed to seek punishment as a way to get attention. In and out of trouble from an early age. In and out of hospitals for his drinking and, later, heroin addiction. In and out of prison.

There was really no surprise about the way Mike turned out. He never had a chance. Never. He had the genes, he had the family history, he had the environmental stress. He died in his 40s of a heroin overdose.

My brother Gary's addiction did surprise me. He was the cutest blond-haired, brown-eyed little kid. He was a year or so younger than me, and his role was being the baby. How could this sensitive boy turn into an addict? He hung out with a bunch of punks in high school, but they were younger than me, and I thought of them as kids—how bad could they be? How much trouble could they get into?

I found out one awful night when I was in the bathroom drying off after a shower. I heard him and his buddies in the bathroom of the apartment upstairs where they lived, talking about a needle. Their voices floated clearly down to me as I heard my baby brother say, "Give me the needle. Give me the fucking *needle!*" I felt like I'd been slammed in the stomach with a battering ram.

At 18, he was doing heroin too.

It was the beginning of a long end for him. I relearned with my brother Gary that you can't help someone when they don't want it. I begged, screamed, reasoned, but got nowhere trying to help him give it up.

He wound up in various institutions, too, and did give up heroin. But he had a lifelong struggle with alcohol.

Gary died 10 months after Mike, from alcohol poisoning. He was 42.

Returning to the present, I put my arm around my daughter, hug her to me. She hugs back, puts her head on my shoulder.

After the lecture, Carolyn and I talk once again until it's time for her to leave.

I run into Diane at the nurses' station. She'll be doing my Duffy again today.

"Soon," she replies to my question of when.

I'm so anxious to get this over with. I hover around the nurses' station talking with some other patients until Diane comes for me. She leads me to the treatment room.

I remove my glasses, put them in their case, and we begin.

While she prepares the emetic drug, I examine my face in the mirror. My hair is already messy, my eyes still puffy, my complexion spotty.

I chug the slimy, bitter medicine. The salt she added has floated to the bottom of the glass. We wait the eight minutes while she sets up my drinks.

"Today we have gin, vodka, white wine, red wine, tequila, and we'll end with gin again."

Oh my God—I'm sick just thinking about it. My upper lip is curling, my nose crinkling.

"Does anyone actually finish all this stuff?" Last time I could get down only a portion of what was put in front of me.

"You'd be surprised. Sometimes the frailest-looking ladies come in and belt them all down, and then the biggest guys come in and can't swallow more than one. You can never tell who's going to do what."

I begin chugging. The gin still doesn't smell bad to me, but drinking it mixed with water is disgusting.

I guzzle one, two, three glasses. Again she tells me that if I don't do something soon, I'll have to help it along. After the fourth, she hands me a tongue depressor and says, "Bring it up."

I put the stick down my throat and throw up.

"Do it again," she directs.

I vomit, spew, gush, puke. I get seven glasses down—all the gin and vodka. My stomach muscles are screaming from the unaccustomed exercise.

I'm wondering how I'll ever get the wine down when she tells me all I have to do with the wine and the tequila is smell, swish, and spit. I practically slobber (well, actually, I *do* slobber) with gratitude.

The white wine is not attractive after all that hard stuff. Coming on its heels, the red wine just about does me in.

Next comes the tequila.

By now, the mixture in the basin looks foul. Smells foul. Retch!

"Your treatment ends at one today," Diane says as she walks me back to my room. She stays to my inside, protecting me from the eyes of the patients and staff at the nurses' station. But I've learned that even if they meet your eyes, it's only for a brief second as they respectfully lower theirs.

"Do I have to have a butterfly today?"

"Oh, yes. They'll be in at 10:30 to give it to you."

I climb into bed, pull the covers over me. Lie down on my back while she tapes the time to my nightstand and positions the disgusting gin-soaked rag next to my pillow.

I throw up several times, lay back panting, exhausted, hurting. A nurse checks on me, asks how many times I've thrown up.

"Any diarrhea?"

"Not yet, but I have a headache."

She returns with my butterfly and an ice pack for my head. I sit up to drink the butterfly. It takes me several seconds to get past the smell of the beer, but I get it down. I lie back down, holding the ice pack to my forehead.

The taste in my mouth is sickening. Right now the overwhelming taste is beer, but I can still taste the red wine and the slimy Emetine. I start to cry, try to hold it back—I know it'll make my head hurt worse, increase the stuffiness in my nose and ears. For a few minutes, though, I can't help myself—I sob uncontrollably until I can once again pull myself together.

"This will all be over by 1," I console myself.

I throw up only once more before the nurse comes in to release me, but I'm still nauseated.

I grab some saltines and head down to the dining room. My stomach is still unsettled, unlike after the first two Duffys, when I felt okay once I was released. I eat a peanut butter cookie and half a sandwich, then go back to my room to rest.

I sleep for about an hour, wake up still queasy. I head out for some fresh air on the deck.

My cell phone indicates both my boys have called. I listen to their messages. Both said, "I love you, Mom, and hope you're doing okay."

I call Mike and break down on the phone. My defenses are gone; I feel lousy physically. Emotionally, I'm spent from dredging up painful memories.

I tell him I hit the wall today. I apologize for crying. He says it's okay, but I know the few times when my mother cried in emotional pain in front of me, it was a painful, traumatic event. I apologize again.

"I love you, Mom, and if this is going to help you get well, hang in there."

We hang up.

The overhead speaker informs us that the video on depression will begin in about 10 minutes. Perfect timing for me—I'm so depressed right now.

Ten minutes into the video, however, I have to leave. I'm still feeling sick. I pass by Diane, mention it to her.

"That's too long. Ask the nurse to give you something."

So I do. Five minutes later, she gives me a shot and the

nausea disappears. I fall asleep peacefully and wake at 6, feeling lots better.

Dinner was at 5, so I scurry to the dining room. I pass Chet on the stairs. He had his treatment around 1:30, but it's after 6 and he's still feeling nauseated. I tell him about my shot and encourage him to ask the nurse for something.

"What do you need, sweetheart?" the cafeteria worker asks me.

"Dinner." I haven't eaten very much all day.

Dinner is spaghetti with meat sauce—my favorite food. And salad. I eat like this is my last meal. I thank the staff profusely and leave.

Tonight's movie is "When a Man Loves a Woman" starring Meg Ryan. I watch for a little while. Meg's character is becoming a drunk. Not too interested, I leave for the food cart, which attracts me so much more.

I hurry to my room with my stash: a tuna sandwich, a ham and cheese, and a dessert. Eat one sandwich, save one for later. Pacing myself with my food as I was never able to do with alcohol. Have two cups of tea. Wonderful, soothing, life-supporting tea.

It's now after 10 as I write in my journal. I did not enjoy today. But I have three of these throw-up treatments down, only (only!) two more to go.

Tomorrow is a rehabilitation interview—a stress-free day. I sleep peacefully.

DAY SIX

Vitals are 98.7, 111/74, 84. Weight 162. I have no Duffy today—I'm happy, celebrating the easy day to come.

I shower, check in at the nurses' station. As I head back to my room, Ruby is making her rounds, clacking down the hall, tapping on each patient's door, chirping, "Good morning, good morning!"

She brings a smile to my face.

In the auditorium awaiting the day's lecture, I again notice the women seated in pairs. I sit in front of Chet. We exchange pleasantries and a high five:

"No Duffy today!"

The topic for today is: "Physical Consequences of Alcoholic Drinking". Dr. Smith begins in his soft voice, telling us how alcohol damages every system in the body, some of them are more forgiving than others.

SYSTEMS MOST AFFECTED BY ALCOHOL

Cardiovascular (heart and blood vessels): Frequently drinking large quantities of alcohol tends to cause elevations in blood fats (lipids). Elevation of the lipids (cholesterol and triglycerides) leads to hardening of the arteries. This hardening (atherosclerosis) is a risk factor in heart attacks and strokes. Alcoholics are at a higher risk for cardiovascular disease than non-drug users.

I've got elevations of both.

Nervous system (brain, spinal cord, various nerves running to all parts of the body): Dead brain cells and other nerve tissues have no power of regeneration, although injured brain cells will regenerate with time and abstinence.

Fortunately, humans have a big reserve, and we don't usually use anywhere near the 100 billion or so brain cells we have. As we age, our brain cells die normally. Usually there is no problem. But if we use them faster than normal due to alcohol, we run out of reserves, and our brain function becomes less than optimal earlier. Short-term memory becomes impaired, arithmetical and other mental manipulation slow, become inaccurate. A progressive type of brain damage occurs that in later stages becomes so extensive it is irreversible.

The good news is that even if the brain and nerve cells are damaged and not functioning properly, if they're not actually dead the cells can, and frequently will, function normally once the drinking stops.

Gastrointestinal system (includes among other things the pancreas, stomach, esophagus, throat, and liver. The liver is the most "prominent organ of injury"): The liver is far more forgiving than the brain. With abstinence, it will most likely return to normal functioning.

The past 10 years of drinking have wrecked my body. I have esophageal reflux, abdominal bloating, diverticulitis, constipation, diarrhea, gas. My tongue is painful, and my mouth frequently breaks out in canker sores. And those are just the things I'm aware of—who knows what else is lurking in my body?

But I'm pretty smug about my liver because all my liver tests have come back normal.

Smug until his next statement: "Don't feel just because

your liver functions are normal your liver is perfect. It merely means you have at least a quarter of a liver functioning normally. On the other hand, abnormal liver tests don't mean you're doomed—it means it has been fatty infiltrated; your liver is enlarged. It will heal if you get off the drug you're using. Even the early stages of cirrhosis are completely reversible."

Dr. Smith summarizes his three-day lecture series by telling us alcoholism is a disease that in many cases appears to be a genetically transmitted biochemical defect. In other cases, it appears to be caused by repeated episodes of heavy drinking bombarding the body's physiology, resulting in the inability to handle alcohol normally.

The disease may be aggravated by psychological and/or social pressures and is characterized by a typical progression of drinking behavior that requires an average of 12 1/2 years of drinking to reach fully developed, overt symptoms and an average of 18 years to reach the stage of deterioration.

At the nurses' station, I ask for my medication for my rehabilitation treatment. My voice is hoarse and raspy. I have a headache left over from yesterday, vague pains in my intestines, persistent low back pain. I have various other aches and pains throughout my body. My ear is stuffed.

I return to my room and fall asleep until I hear: "Wake up! Time for your sedation treatment."

I'm brought to the treatment room, the IV is started. The counselor, Todd, asks me to read my affirmations after he reviews them with me.

I read a few, then—just as before—wake up when the session is over.

Question: "On a scale of 1 to 10, 1 being weak and 10 being

strong, what is your current level of aversion to alcohol or drugs you are treating for?"

Response: "4." Still a 4 on a scale of 1 to 10? How many Duffys will it take to get to a 10?

Question: "How has alcohol or other drugs kept you from achieving your goals?"

Response: "I get to a place where I am happy, then I drink. I feel like I am in a circle that revolves around alcohol and I sabotage myself."

Why do I sabotage myself, I wonder. I've always been afraid of failure. Am I equally or more afraid of success?

There were several other questions, none of which surprised me. They had to do with what I'll do for recreation when I leave the hospital, how I will deal with stress.

My favorite question and response is this:

Question: "What will be great in your life without using alcohol or drugs?"

I answer: "Being alive... appreciating the small things in life, tapping into creativity that now has alcohol barriers around it..."

My subconscious has been honing my career vision. I tell them I want to write a book about my experience here and become an alcohol and nutrition counselor.

The question and response that surprised and pleased me was this:

Question: "Do you see your chemical dependency as a disease or as a function of poor willpower?"

Response: "I have a disease."

This is a breakthrough for me. I've been beating myself up for years for what I perceived as my weaknesses, moral flaws, my "bad" character. Now I'm accepting myself on a subconscious as well as conscious level for what I am. And what I have.

I didn't want to see this as a disease because I didn't want to use that as an excuse for my drinking. I'd been listening to too many people who think of alcoholism as a personality defect. But looking at that logic now, it strikes me as ironic.

What's worse: being genetically damaged or having no willpower? To me, having a disease is much worse. Being able to pass something like this down to your kids is horrific. Who would want to think about this as a disease if it wasn't?

And who needs an excuse to drink anyway?

I'm wheeled back to my room. And although I'd like to sleep some more, it's 12:10—lunchtime!

Lunch today is a taco salad in the shell. The shell is baked, not greasy, and the entire thing is wonderful. I sit with one of the women pairs—Barbara and Debbie—and Jerry, who is going home tomorrow. Debbie talks about a 21-day treatment program she'd been through and relapsed. Barbara and Debbie giggle a lot. Bonded.

After lunch, I head for the deck. The weather over the past week has been spectacular: clear, deep blue skies, bright sun, fresh air. Today I appreciate being alive!

The deck overlooks a pretty rockery wall planted with a variety of flowers, shrubs, and trees. A gardener works to keep everything neat.

The gentleman with the walker sits quietly. I introduce myself.

"My name is Alan," he tells me in a heavily accented voice. A shy smile starts with his lips, meets his warm brown eyes.

We talk a little bit. He tells me he is part Comanche,

part Kiowa, He shares some details of his early life—pretty sad—until he was adopted and brought up by the Navaho tribe in Arizona. He needed to share, and I needed to listen. And I remember thinking, "Man, whenever you think you have it bad..."

When I get up to go take a nap, we hug.

Back in my room, I'm ready to drop off to sleep when Dr. Smith stops in during his rounds. "Your chart indicates you are doing well," he says.

"What in your chart tells you that?"

"Your counter-conditioning level being a 4 at this point in your treatment."

So, even though I was worried about it being only a 4, he is quite pleased with my progress!

It's 4 p.m. The mandatory discussion is entitled "Communication" and is given by Fred. He tells us it's about communicating with ourselves, and he passes out several handouts. One is entitled "How to Do Nothing."

HOW TO DO NOTHING

At least once during the day, take five or 10 minutes to sit quietly and do nothing. Focus on the sounds around you, your emotions, and any tension in your body. Sitting quietly slows heart rate and reduces blood pressure. It can also change your perspective and increase your control over events.

Studies show that the most stressful situations are things we can't control.

We can't change the past. We can't predict or change the future. The only thing any of us can control is the present moment. When people practice doing nothing, they regain a sense of control and ease stress.

Fred tells us that this is one of the hardest things for many people to do because we're used to thinking of our worth in terms of what we get done.

Then we all practice doing nothing while sitting in our chairs.

It is hard!

Another handout is entitled "18 Posture Chi Kung." Chi Kung is the art of developing vital energy for health, vitality, mind expansion, and spiritual cultivation. We practice several of the exercises on the handout.

Today's discussion is more philosophical than what we've had so far. Fred passes out an Irish poem; one of the lines is "May there always be work for your hands to do."

I think this is pretty ironic considering the first exercise today was how to do nothing.

There's a new patient in the audience today, and after the lecture several of us stop to introduce ourselves. His name is Ken. We've seen him power walking around the halls and grounds all day today. We fill him in: how and when to get his vitamins, check his treatment schedules, etc. We look at his schedule for tomorrow—he is scheduled for both a Duffy and Faradic therapy. I'm wondering why he rates both treatments, but I personally don't want to find out. We give him some more advice and go down to dinner.

Dinner is ham, scalloped potatoes, fresh rolls, salad, fresh peaches with cream. I sit at a table of women—Barbara, Debbie, Glenda, and Myra—and we jabber away, mostly about what we told people about where we are: anywhere but here.

On to tonight's movie: "Bagger Vance". Again, I'm not interested. I leave to hit the food cart. It's not there yet, so I sit in my room with the door open, waiting, waiting, waiting with such impatience. As though I've never eaten before. I check three times and it's still not there.

"Snacks!" calls Sam, hurrying past my room. He can see the food cart from his. I scurry up, grab two egg salad sandwiches, five olives, five cookies, then return to my lair clutching the items to my chest.

I gobble, write, read a little "Mutant". It's the story of an American doctor who gets invited by an Australian agency to live and work in Australia for a few years. She begins to study and treat half-Aborigines in an urban setting. She is exposed to government propaganda that maintains Australia was empty when the Brits settled it, that however the Aborigines got there, they were an inferior species who don't feel pain as the "higher" humans do; they're basically lazy, etc.

Still confused as to what this has to do with me, I read on.

The doctor gets invited to do a walkabout with the Aborigines across the desert. She's learning their customs, their incredible stamina, their oral history. Who they really are. Which differs significantly from the government propaganda.

All I can come up with that pertains to me is that Gary, my counselor, might want to demonstrate how different interpretations of the same events influence our behaviors, thoughts, and actions.

I'm done reading for the day. It's bedtime.

DAY SEVEN

6:15 a.m. Vitals: 97.6, 91/59, 70. Weight 163.

I had an unsettling dream last night. Too real: I'm setting up to get drunk: planning the day, planning the excuses that will enable me to get into the bedroom alone with my bottle(s), planning my excuses for after. Writing them down so I can remember to whom I told what.

In my wakened state, I say aloud, "No, I'm never going to do that anymore." But the fact that I'm dreaming it frightens me, and I need to talk this over with a counselor.

Lying back, I think about the Duffy today. I can't eat, only drink fluids. I don't feel like getting up yet. I'm so tired. I decide to meditate, but I'm having a hard time. I'm not sure I even know how. So I try to focus instead on what I'm grateful for today.

Today I'm grateful to be alive, to be sober, to be here, even though "here" is going to make me throw up today. I'm grateful that I have a husband who, though I don't think he understands my problem, has supported me through various attempts to get better. Has never belittled me for my drinking.

I'm grateful I have three terrific kids who are each supporting me in his or her own way. Whom I love more than anything, and who (I realize now) appear to not only love me, but like me too. They actually want to spend time with me!

I'm grateful to have the support of the friends who know I'm here, who have called to ask how I'm doing, sending their support and love.

I'm grateful to have a good relationship now with my 85-year-old mother.

Our relationship changed a lot over the years. Somewhere along the line, our roles got reversed—I tried to take care of her. I became the good girl of the family (at least until high school) and did everything right so as not to contribute to her unhappiness or pain. But in doing this, I took on those unhappy things, those painful things, and they made me physically sick in many ways: constipation so bad sometimes I could hardly stand up; stomach upset so bad sometimes I could hardly eat. Nonexistent self-esteem.

Later, I remember being angry and bitter at her for not leaving my father when he was at his abusive worst. Didn't she care about us?

Angry and tormented when she didn't have my brothers arrested when they stole her blind, opening up charge cards in her name, buying thousands of dollars worth of stuff to sell so they could get their drugs.

Furious when she went into debt to pay for their crimes. Unbelievably hurt at her hurt, her pain, and not able to do anything about it.

Hurt, frustrated, angry, sick. Stuffed inside myself.

Finally, after I got married, I "divorced" my family for self-preservation. I couldn't stand to talk with my two addicted brothers. I had so much anger towards them. I couldn't stand to listen to my mother tell me about their latest escapades or hospitalizations or her visits to the prisons or the institutions wherever they currently were.

So I'd talk to her once every two weeks or so just to let her know I was still alive. I had moved with my husband about 90 miles away. She couldn't visit because of what my brothers would (and did) do to her house and with her possessions while she was gone. She was basically a prisoner to their addictions.

A prisoner, but at the same time their nursemaid. No prison was too far, no institution too scary for her not to visit. Me? I lived 90 miles away. I didn't get visits. When my first child was born, she came and spent one night with me. And that was only because I asked.

I was bitter. I missed her not being a part of my kids' early lives. I hurt so much, and got angrier that she put my brothers ahead of me.

When my two brothers died in the same year, I became much more available to her. And she was free to have a relationship with me.

She began visiting me more often, bringing lots of homemade food – meatloaf, pot roast with homemade mashed potatoes, vegetable soup. This is and has always been my mother's primary way of showing love. Maybe that's why I love food so much.

But it hasn't always been easy these past 11 years.

Sometimes we have that love-hate relationship thing going on. Sometimes I think she's jealous of me and she says hurtful things. But I've learned a lot, try to accept our relationship for what it is, and try not to contradict her when her selective memory enables her to make an outrageous statement about how close a family we were growing up. I have to remind myself that she's 85, and anything I say now would have no point except to hurt.

I decide to call her (it's now 9:45 a.m. on the East Coast where she lives).

She doesn't know I'm here, and I won't tell her. Today is her regular day to be with "the ladies." Each week they alternate treating each other to lunch. I'm hoping it's her turn to feed them because she'll be in a hurry and won't be able to talk long. I'm worried there'll be an announcement over the loudspeaker, sparking her curiosity about where I'm calling from.

When the other ladies take their turn treating, they generally get a bucket of chicken or a pizza or go to the nearest hot dog stand. Not my mother. She is recuperating from knee replacement surgery, bent over with osteoporosis, her right arm half useless from rotator cuff tears. She now has to hold pots with two hands, and she can no longer pick up a whole chicken—it's too heavy.

She still cooks up a storm. But now she has to start on Tuesday or Wednesday to make Thursday lunch.

Today is not her day to cook, so she has lots of time to talk.

I tell her I'm at the mall so I'm covered if a voice does come over the loudspeaker. She's always confused about the time change, so she doesn't realize it's only 6:45 a.m. where I am.

We talk for a while about the computer I recently set up for her. As we do, the nurse walks in with my morning medication. Putting out my hand to silence her, I say, "Gotta go, Mom, they're ready to ring me up."

I apologize to the nurse, explain to her that my mother doesn't know I'm here.

"No problem," she says. I take my meds and she leaves.

Breakfast arrives—my Duffy breakfast: hot water, low-sodium beef bouillon packet, mystery jello. I'm never having that low-sodium bouillon again. I'm desperate enough to eat the jello, though. Oops, there's no spoon.

I head off to the snack area to get one. Chet and Jerry are talking in the hall. Ken practically jogs by.

"Ken!" Jerry calls, "we've taken a poll. You've got to stop the walking. You're making the rest of us look bad!"

We all laugh. Ken stops to talk for a minute or two, then resumes his power walking.

"Are you leaving today, Jerry?" I ask.

Jerry has asked a few questions in our various lectures, and it seems he is hiding behind a wall of sarcasm. When he answers yes, I ask him how he feels about going home.

"Well, I'll never take another drink of Emetine—I've developed quite an aversion to it," he quips.

"You mentioned the other night at the meeting your feelings of being alone. Can I give you my phone number to call if you just need to hear a voice?"

"Yes," he replied, "that would be good."

I can't tell from his face whether or not my gesture is accepted in the spirit in which it was given, but it's there for the taking. Or not. I write down my number.

Chet and I compare notes. We are both getting Duffys today. His is in the afternoon; mine is scheduled for the morning. Diane tells me it will be at 8:45.

Myra walks by and joins the conversation.

She came in several days ago and has been detoxing ever since. She has medium-brown hair, sharp chin, nose. Pouches of fluid underneath her eyes, which can be seen behind her glasses. She's about 5 feet 6 inches and very thin. Very smart. Very personable.

"Myra, what do you have planned for today?" I ask.

"Today I get to throw up!" she says excitedly.

"Welcome to the club!" I shout, hugging her. She fiercely clutches me back, thanking me. Who would have ever thought this would be a club people would be happy to join?

We all grab pitchers of fluids, head down around 8 to see the obligatory video on "Enabling". A Father Martin from AA is the video's lecturer. I can hardly concentrate because I'm worrying whether I'll have time to get enough fluid into my body before I'm called for my Duffy.

But some of his remarks do make it through: How the best way to help alcoholics is to let them face the consequences of their drinking. When you pay their bills or make excuses to their boss or others, you are freeing them, enabling them to take their next drink. Stop doing that, he tells us.

My first thought is: "Are you kidding?" I have such mixed emotions over this issue.

I think back to my childhood and know that if we didn't make excuses for my father—yes, he would have faced the consequences—he would have lost his job. But we would have suffered along with him. We would have been left with no income instead of the income we got after he was done drinking his portion of it. We would have lost our house. We came close enough as it was.

How can a mother not tell her husband's boss a lie when the alternative means her children will suffer even more?

Yet, growing up I was so angry with my mother for not leaving my father, thinking: "How could she love us and still stay here?"

Those were the days when my mother worked as a housecleaner for $5.00 a day, or in a paper goods factory for not much more.

Those, too, were the days when we'd occasionally have our electricity shut off because we had no money. I'm sure my mother wondered how could we possibly survive on one salary when we barely survived on two. She probably felt as trapped as we did, but those were also the days when most women did not leave their husbands, no matter what.

Enabling, codependency is not a black-and-white issue.

"It is not your disease. It's the alcoholic's disease," Father Martin continues.

Disease. There's that word again.

I think part of the reason I've been afraid to see this as a disease is that I wouldn't know what to do with my anger and disappointment toward my father and brothers. All sorts of uncomfortable feelings awaken in me. Growing up, I alternately scorned and pitied them—weaklings who couldn't give up booze and drugs even when their families and their lives were at stake. No willpower.

Whatever I have, I realize I have a lot of thinking to do.

First, my father. I hated him for the pain he caused us. Was terrified of his mercurial temper. Was mortified by his behavior. But he tried to control his drinking—he attended AA meetings at various times, and I know he went into detox treatment several times while I was growing up. Sometimes he stayed sober a long time afterward, other times only a few days. I imagine talking with him:

"Dad, what did you talk about in AA? Did you express guilt, shame, powerlessness? Did it hurt you knowing you were hurting your kids and your wife? Did you ever cry? I'm sorry you never beat your addiction. I'm sorry for what you had to go through. I'm sorry for what you put us through. I know you loved me."

Visualizing my father crying really gets to me. I'm sitting in the auditorium watching the video and tears are pouring down my face. And I realize my story is being rewritten.

When the video ends, I'm called for my treatment. Diane is once again my nurse. There is another nurse, Debbie, here at the hospital, but so far I haven't seen her. I'm happy to see Diane; I'm feeling comfortable with her now.

I tell her I'm almost ill just walking into the room. Today is supposed to be a lot of glasses. A LOT of glasses! I discuss the last treatment and the butterfly that never came back up.

"You won't get a butterfly today—you don't need it."

I don't know who made that decision, but I'm not going to argue.

I drink my two glasses of the emetic drug. It's really hard to get them down—I'm practically gagging already, my throat closing in protest.

Some patients have told me that you can have a picture taken in the Duffy room to help with your relapse prevention. While we wait for the drug to take effect, I request one. I tell Diane I don't need an action shot.

I also don't need to pose. In the photo I look haggard, sick.

She pours the gin. Adds water. I get halfway through the first glass and I start puking. I shudder, spit. I get a headache.

I get the rest of that first glass down, maybe one more. I'm throwing up so often that Diane tells me I don't have to swallow—just smell, swish, and spit.

Today whiskey is added to the mix. The smell, swish, and spit part of the treatment goes by very quickly, and I'm whisked back to my room. Diane gives me an ice bag for my head.

I lie down. Throw up. Lie back down. Pull the blankets up. I'm cold. Then hot, so hot. I lay back, panting, the ice bag across my forehead, eyes closed. My stomach begins gurgling, and I know what that means.

I make it to the bathroom. Stumble back to bed.

"What's your nausea level?" my nurse asks.

"It's a 2, and I have wicked diarrhea."

It's 10:10 a.m. Two hours to go. The sign with the time is taped to my nightstand and my mantra continues: "This will all be over by 12:10."

Another bout of diarrhea and vomiting. I wash my hands, return to bed. The muscles in the side of my throat hurt. My head pounds.

Finally I'm done. I've given it all up. I have nothing left. I am spent emotionally and physically.

I can't even cry.

The lunch announcement is made. I'm slightly nauseated and have a headache. But I'm hungry! How can that be?

Lunch is homemade pea soup and ham sandwiches. I manage to eat about half before I need to rest.

I try to nap. My son Craig calls and we talk. He tells me he loves me. I sleep, hoping my headache and remaining nausea will go away. I miss the mandatory afternoon lecture on boundaries and self-esteem.

I don't wake up until dinner. How important meals are around here. They structure your day, give you something to look forward to.

Tonight I sit at a table with Glenda and Sharon, another female pair that has formed. Glenda is in her 40s—a tiny, attractive, blue-eyed blonde. She appears timid. Sharon is in her early 30s—medium height and weight. Beautiful, huge, dark blue eyes with large pupils. Her hair is dirty blond, long, styled. She is gorgeous.

This is when I learn why the women have formed groups: they room together! I forgot there even were semiprivate rooms here. There are only three other patient rooms in my wing, and they're all private. One is occupied by Chet, one by Sam, one by Mary.

Not so the other wings. They are mostly semiprivate. The women room together, so they sit at meals together, go to presentations together, hang out on the deck. I'm so relieved to realize that I'm wandering around by myself not because I'm unlikable, but because of our physical circumstances.

And, of course, because I'm so independent.

As I return to my room, Chet emerges from his on his way to dinner.

"Bumpy road" is all he says, not looking too good. But, like the rest of us, he won't miss a meal if he can help it.

Tonight's optional movie is "Clean and Sober". I opt not to go. The week is really catching up with me. I am so tired, but I head out to the deck for some fresh air. As I pass the nurses' station, I see a new guy who I first noticed last night, pacing up and down the hall, mumbling angrily. He stops at the nurses' station, where they put up with none of his lip.

I head back to my room to write some more.

DAY EIGHT

Today's a rehabilitation interview day! No Duffy!
Vitals are 97.3, 140/81, 79. Weight 160.
I run into Chet and Myra at the scale at 6:30 a.m. We are all so excited not to be having Duffys. We stand and talk about Chet's rough times.

"Well," he says, "I came in and told them to give me all they've got. And they sure are doing that. But I can take it," he adds.

Myra says she's been drinking for 25 years times 365 days—she can handle five Duffy treatments. She has her second one today. "But I'm not drinking anything of color anymore before my treatments."

We all laugh. Throwing up in color is so disgusting!

I shower, wash and style my hair. Put on makeup, contact lenses. Once again I run into Chet, who has been out power walking with Ken.

I show him my picture taken in the Duffy room. He doesn't want one.

"I hope to put all this behind me. I don't want any reminders.

We talk about attending meetings after we're done. He's not interested. He doesn't like AA. "Too much ceremony. Too many war stories."

He wonders if he just hasn't found the right AA meeting. He's been to about six different ones. I tell him the Monday night meeting here worked for me and ask him to give it a chance.

We talk about ourselves a little. I tell him how independent I've always been.

"I've always been independent too," adds Chet.

But we're learning that there's a difference between being independent and isolating ourselves. I'm going to try to reach out more. I've already started to do that here, with Chet and Myra.

I'm gaining confidence. Once again, I think of my family and friends. They wouldn't love me, or like me, if I wasn't deserving.

I think.

As I write this in my journal, I realize that I'm getting excited about life after treatment. I want to set some goals.

I used to be a goal-oriented person. Looking to the future was my best coping mechanism. It took the anxiety from the present, made me forget the pain of the past, at least for a while.

Once I figured out the goal, I planned for it, went after it. When I was younger, figuring out my goals was easy—there were so many: go to college, get a good job, graduate college, get married, buy a house, have kids, raise the kids.

But the past few years, I've had no goals. I haven't been able to think of anything I really wanted to aim for. Is it due to empty-nest syndrome? Alcohol? Midlife crisis? Boredom? All of the above? For me, living without goals has been a sad and pointless existence—for one thing, because I have nothing to look forward to—for another, because I don't know how to just be.

I shared this inability once with my counselor. She told me this is often the point—when the kids leave home and you reach a certain age—when problem drinkers break through the barrier to become uncontrolled alcoholics. They think they have nothing to look forward to. If they're lucky, they start seeing counselors, get their disease under control, and their goal becomes getting mentally and physically healthy, some for the first time ever.

So now I'm thinking, "How great is this? I want to set some goals."

I want to publish my journal—I want to bring up and out all the stuff I've been living with forever. I want to put words on paper so they no longer have the power to hurt me.

I want to share my experience with others.

I want to do something that benefits others.

I want to learn to just be.

I can't eat breakfast today, so I talk with John, the admissions counselor. I ask about confidentiality, what I signed when I was admitted. I don't want to violate any confidentiality rules if and when I publish my journal.

He tells me the confidentiality is all on the part of the Hospital, and I am free to write what I please as long as I don't violate any other patient's privacy. Author's note: I changed even the first names of patients I refer to here (the staff's names, however, are real).

Today's video is "Portrait of Addiction", produced by Bill Moyers. It's about six people, all of whom had addictions, all of whom beat them. They came from various walks of life. No one is immune—be it the middle-aged, middle-class white female, the teenager who starts to drink because of peer pressure, the young career guy snorting coke, the ghetto heroin addict.

When the film is over, I return to my room, passing Mary's.

"Hi Mary," I call. "Can I get you anything?"
She shakes her head.

Yolanda, my rehab interview nurse, pops into my room to tell me the treatment will be given in my room today. That's okay with me. I'm quite comfy in my bed.

A young Asian woman walks in, puts her computer on my nightstand, takes a seat. "I'm Ahn, a counselor trainee," she says.

Ahn, like Judy and Todd before her, is impressed that I've written out all my own affirmations. I guess it's not done too often—I know some of the patients haven't even read their packets yet, even though it's been stressed over and over. That makes me sad, because affirmations are so powerful. And to get a chance to put them right into your subconscious is an opportunity of a lifetime.

"Are you a writer?" Yolanda asks.

"Why do you ask?" I say, fascinated by her question. I love writing. Growing up, I always wanted to write a book and I always knew it would be about alcoholism and drugs—about my father and my brothers, of course.

Never, *never* did I dream I would be the alcoholic main character.

"I don't know why," she says. "But the first day I met you and you started speaking, that's the impression I got.

I smile hugely. "Well, Yolanda, that's what I'm setting as my goal. To write a best seller and to be on 'Oprah'!"

She laughs and tells me she'll get my autograph before I become too famous.

I laugh too, but I'm serious. And I'm filled with joy that I have enough confidence to say these things out loud.

After the IV is inserted, Ahn asks me to read my affirmations. Once again I get to about six: "I respond peacefully to any and all stressful situations in life."

I awake around 11 a.m., nurses and equipment gone. I feel great! Tired, but great!

The first question: "On a scale of 1 to 10, 1 being weak and 10 being strong, what is your current level of counter-conditioning to alcohol?"

My response: 7 or 8!

Question: I'm asked under what circumstances I would be most likely to relapse.

My answer: "If I don't eat right, sleep right, and get the support I need from my husband."

I talk to Gary, tell him that under sedation I identified him as an obstacle to my recovery.

He already knows this, and he takes responsibility for his part in our troubled relationship. He knows I've been furious with him, hurt by his sometimes scornful disrespect. He says things will change; I hope so. He knows I won't let him disrespect me anymore. I'm going through hell to change, and I hope he'll make an effort too.

While talking with Gary, I realize I am feeling more positive toward him; I have faith that he will try. I'm optimistic about our relationship now that we've got all the cards on the table.

Lunch isn't until 12, so I have two cups of life-restoring tea. Wonderful tea. It never tasted better.

I return a call from my son, Craig, who had left a message yesterday wanting to know if he needed to hop a plane and come rescue me. "I'm doing great, Craig," I tell him. "I hit the wall the other day, but I'm doing great now. Making plans, looking forward to life. And I don't have to throw up today. Doesn't get any better than this!"

We give each other our love.

As I hang up, I think about how often my kids and I tell each other "I love you." There's not a conversation, not an e-mail, that we don't express it. How different from my family when I was growing up.

My mother is a very reserved person. Intimacy frightens her. When you hug her, she gets all embarrassed and instead of hugging you straight on, she pushes you into her armpit so the amount of touching is minimal. For years, she signed her cards to my husband: "Take Care, from Mrs.G."

Growing up, I can't remember my mother saying "I love you" to me or to anyone else. I do remember the first time a few years ago when I said it to her. I thought about it for months, tried to sneak it in when the words wouldn't stand there all by themselves and die from loneliness. Or rejection.

Finally I thought the time was right. One day we were on the phone. As she was about to hang up, I said, "I love you, Mom."

Pause.

Pregnant pause.

"You too," she said quickly. And hung up.

Since then, I tell her occasionally. And once as she was hanging up, without any prompting, she said to me, "Love ya." Which to me seems less intimate than "I love you". But it's definitely progress!

I'm feeling good, so I call my friend Nancy, who knows where I am. She and I are a lot alike: both half Irish, both from a family with a lot of brothers, both with alcoholic fathers. I can tell Nancy anything, so I tell her about my bowel movements. I know she'll want to hear.

"I'm honored that you're sharing this with me," she laughs.

Lunchtime! Afterwards, I head out to walk. Not walk, walk, walk like Ken, but to explore, get some fresh air, enjoy the beautiful day.

I'm feeling so good today. It's Friday, 12:30. I'll be done with my treatment by this time Sunday. I'm on the home stretch.

I keep adding to my list of things to do when I get out:

Get a massage. Regularly.
Find a whole-grains cooking class.
Develop a relapse prevention packet.
Learn a lot more about nutrition and recovery.
Publish my journal.

I think about going back to work when I get out. My boss expects me back next Thursday, but I know it's critical for me to develop a basic pattern for my sobriety. Eating right, exercising, cooking the right foods, getting into good habits. I decide to go for broke and take a few more days off.

After my walk, I sit on the deck to journal. The gardener is again working. Ken is *walking*. Alan sits quietly with his walker. Other patients sit on the deck, smoking, talking. It's become quite comfortable now. Family.

I run into my counselor, Gary, on the way to afternoon class. Thinking there must be a "right" answer to what I'm supposed to take away from the book he loaned me (and that I'm gonna get that answer!), I eagerly ask him if he is trying to get me to understand something about life seen from different perspectives.

"You remember we spoke about truth the other day?

What is truth? The British version or the Aborigines' version?"

As I walk away I wonder: "What is *my* truth?"

Today's mandatory class is "Support Groups," led by Fred. We get handouts on many different options. We talk about how we might like each one. In addition to AA and those meetings held at Schick Shadel, there are others.

Here are a few we talked about:

Women for Sobriety: www.womenforsobriety.org/

SOS-Secular Organization for Sobriety. www. unhooked.com. "Sobriety is achieved without resorting to a Higher Power."

RR-Rational Recovery using AVRT (Addictive Voice Recognition Therapy): www.rational.org

SMART-Self-Management and Recovery Training www.smartrecovery.org

There were lots of groups mentioned, and when I did a search of the Web, I discovered tons more. There seems to be something for almost everyone.

My literature packet is growing with good information.

After the class, I check my schedule for tomorrow's Duffy. My last one!

Diane's not going to be in. "I don't want to start with someone new for my last one!" I whine to myself. But at least my treatment is scheduled for the morning. Thank God—I can't wait to get it over with!

There's a Duffy scheduling hierarchy here. Discharges go first, then recaps, then fifth Duffys, then newer Duffys. This being my fifth Duffy, I'm high on the list, so I should be among the first. Happy about this, I grab a cup of tea and head for the deck.

On the deck, the patient I had seen pacing and mumbling angrily is out there smoking. But today he's talking and laughing. I join the conversation, tell him how good he looks, how nice it is to see him smiling.

He doesn't even remember being so angry – turns out he was detoxing. His brain is clear now—his name is Jim, and he's a crab fisherman in Alaska. We're talking about the few cities in Alaska I've visited when tonight's movie announcement is made.

It's "Stuart Saves His Family" starring Al Franken. I've seen it before. It's a mockumentary on self-help groups. It's hysterical when viewed with a bunch of people—it's the type of movie you like to groan out loud to with others, especially when he says things like "An attitude of gratitude is no platitude." And "I'm good enough, smart enough, and, doggone it, people like me!"

When I leave the auditorium, I again find most of the other patients on the deck: Chet, Myra, Jim, Ken, Vera, Sheila. A group therapy session without a leader.

We talk about our needs, mine being to reach out to other human beings.

We giggle about our treatments and the body products we put out. I'm told there is an antipoop drug I should ask for to control the diarrhea.

Ken, the walker, is sarcastic, cynical about Schick Shadel. This is his third program.

Jim, the crab fisherman, is once again charming.

Vera, a new patient, asks who I am and where I'm located. She's never seen me before. I tell her I'm in kind of a private wing. We talk about the pros and cons of that. The pros: doing my business in private. The cons: I won't come out of the program with as many relationships as those in semiprivate rooms or even in private rooms in a more populated wing.

We talk about exchanging e-mail addresses to keep in touch. Chet and I are thinking ahead to Sunday when we'll be sprung. We joke about getting out of the last Duffy.

I turn in early tonight. I'm beat.

DAY NINE

I wake up at 6. A nurse gives me my meds—this morning two antipoop pills have been added.

"Have a nice day," she smiles.

"Right," I reply silently. I'm in a foul mood this morning. Foul!!! I have a headache. And I'm tired, so tired.

My body has had it. My emotions have had it. I'm crying as Brandon, my nurse, comes in to take my vital signs: 97.2, 106/77, 71. Weight 159.

"Feeling sad today, huh?"

I nod my head yes.

"But it's your last Duffy," he says. "And there are two Duffy ladies on today—Diane was called in because we have so many to do, so you should be able to get it over with early."

My spirits lift a little. Maybe I'll get Diane after all. I tell myself that as soon as my Duffy is over, I can begin my new life.

Brandon returns a short time later with my breakfast tray. Low-sodium bullion and jello.

"Please get that out of here!" I bark loudly, unpleasantly. I can't stand to even look at it.

I put on my robe, sip ice water, journal, resolve to suck it up and get it the hell over with. I'm trying to improve my mood.

Around 8 a.m. I head out to the nurses' station to see if I can get a better idea about my Duffy time. While I'm there, Diane calls Sharon to the treatment room. It's her last one, too. "Good to get it over first thing," she says almost cheerfully, almost skipping into the room.

"That's what I want to do—get it over with. Diane, you know me—I need to know about when I'm due."

"I don't have you on my schedule today. Debbie does."

Just as I feared – I have to end my treatment with someone new. My anxiety level shoots up. I don't know Debbie. Who is she? Diane points her out. I look over at her, talking to Chet, telling him he'll be second up, in about 45 minutes. He smiles at me as he goes back to his room to prepare.

"Hi, Debbie; I'm Kathy. Can you tell me when I'll be treated?"

"I don't know," she replies. "You're scheduled for one-on-one counseling this morning, so they postponed your Duffy until this afternoon. I can't schedule you until you're done with your counseling, which may be as late as 2 or 3 p.m. You should go eat breakfast."

I explode! All of my energy has been focused on getting through the next few hours. My life can't start until I am done with the last Duffy.

I have a meltdown at the nurses' station in front of everyone. I cry, I yell. I throw a tantrum: "I want my Duffy this morning. I have to have my Duffy this morning. I have Duffy seniority!" Like I'm in a Duffy union, for God's sake.

Can't my counselor be scheduled after my treatment?" I snuffle, whine out loud. I know I won't be able to concentrate on what the counselor has to say. I have too much pain, too much emotion. My nerves are frazzled.

"I can't decide that," Debbie responds. "But you can ask your nurse to get in touch with your counselor."

There are many people milling about behind the counter at the nurses' station. No one looks at me as I approach.

"Pay fucking attention to me," I want to shout. "Human being in extreme distress here!"

But I haven't spoken out loud. It takes me a few minutes

to pull myself together, to stop my lips from quivering, the tears from flowing. I ask the first person who looks up to please get me a nurse.

The nurse misunderstands what I'm asking for. "Sometimes they don't do the fifth Duffy, depending on your progress. Sit down here and wait for the doctor."

As I sit there crying in the most public place in the hospital, Chet passes by on his way to the auditorium, unaware of my drama. "Well, Kathleen, what's your schedule for today?" he asks kindly.

I look at him, tears rolling down my face. "Bad morning, Chet. They want me to wait till this afternoon for my Duffy. I can't."

He nods sympathetically. He gets it – he doesn't want to wait for his Duffy either. But he moves on, seeing how upset I am, giving me space.

When I can talk again, I tell the nurse I'm not trying to get out of the Duffy; I just want it scheduled for this morning.

She talks to the counselor, who agrees to see me in the afternoon. I get scheduled third, after Chet. I thank the nurse profusely, then head down to see the morning's video: "The Hijacked Brain", part of the Bill Moyers series.

I'm beyond reason this morning, appalled by my behavior—not able to concentrate too well. But the parts of the video I do see impress me, and I decide to get these videos from the library once I'm out.

Chet is called for his treatment at 8:40. I know I'm next. "Hurry, Chet," I say silently as he passes by my seat, puts his hand on my seat back.

My name is called at 9:10. I pee, head upstairs. The treatment room I'm assigned to today is a mirror image of the other one:

sink on the right, counters on the left. I sit down, apologize to Debbie for being so rude. And then I cry some more.

"It's a tough time," she says. And, repeating what Diane told me, adds: "Lots of things come up here."

Once again, I'm sure she's not referring to just the alcohol.

"Let's get started."

She gives me the emetic drug.

"Your glasses are bigger than Diane's," I whine.

"No, they're not."

"Ick! Did you put salt in this one?"

"Yes."

"Oh no you didn't," I'm thinking. I don't see any little salt particles on the bottom of the glass. But I don't think it's wise for me to pursue this thought out loud.

I can hardly get the bitter shit down.

We wait for the drug to take effect.

"Drink up!"

I guzzle one.

Two.

My throat is starting to close up on three. I pause halfway through, throw up.

Unlike Diane, whose conversation is generally limited to "guzzle" and "breathe," Debbie acts like my personal puke coach.

"Look at yourself in the mirror. That's what you look like when you drink!"

I lift my head, look at my red, haggard face, greasy hair sticking up in all directions.

"Guzzle."

I chug.

Puke!

"Alcohol makes you sick!" Debbie says. "Look at you!"

Retch!!

"You're allergic to alcohol! You can't even stand the taste on your lips!"

Throw up!

Then my headache starts. "My head!" I groan. I've gone through gin, vodka, more gins, tequila. Mostly I'm just spitting it out. My throat is almost closed. My lips are tingling.

"Even the smell is making you sick!" she yells. "You HATE the stuff!"

We both collapse with laughter; mine the kind of hysterical laugh that comes right before you break down helplessly in tears.

I compose myself quickly. "Let's get it over with!"

"The rest you can smell, swish, and spit."

I take one whiff of gin. Retch. I begin a mantra of my own out loud: "Alcohol makes me sick!" Spit.

"I am allergic to alcohol!" Sniff.

"I hate alcohol!" Swish.

"Alcohol makes me sick!!!" Vomit.

When I'm able to move, Debbie escorts me back to my room.

Another brutal wave of nausea. Flopping across the bed, I throw up into the round blue bucket, all the while clutching an ice bag to my aching head. A pair of shoes enters my field of vision. I look up, squinting.

"What?" I croak.

It's Dr. Moran. I lean back down, retch some more.

"Kathleen, dear, I'll stop by later."

"Please," I whimper as he leaves.

The spasm subsides. I fall back onto my side, ice bag gripped against my forehead. The gin-soaked rag sits next to my face—its repulsive fumes wafting up my nose, adding to the nausea. As instructed, I think about my drinking and how I got here.

I have plenty of time to contemplate. I think not only of how I got here but also that I'll never be here again. I'll never need alcohol treatment again because I will never drink again. Never. I know if I do, I'll have to come back here, and I'm not ever gonna come back here!

My treatment ends at 12:10, but I can't move, even for lunch.

When I can finally rise, I head out to the deck with some saltines. It is a spectacular Seattle day: sky deep blue, not a cloud in sight. Bright sun, green leaves and plantings all around. Perfect!

The gardener moves up and down in the rockery. Jim and Myra are talking. I tell him how wonderful it is to see him now. Sober, he is a sweet and charming guy!

It's about 2:30, and I head back to my room to use the bathroom. I haven't seen Chet since he left for his treatment this morning, but I sure have heard him. His door is open, but the sign on it is set to: "No Visitors Please." Since we haven't faithfully been using the signs to indicate our moods, I tap on his door, let him know it's okay to send me away if he doesn't feel like talking.

He comes to the door (we're not allowed to be in the rooms of patients of the opposite sex) and we stand there talking for a while.

"They broke me, Kathleen," he says. "I'm done".

"Me too. I am so glad that was my last Duffy."

"If they had a sixth Duffy, I think I'd be in a cab right now heading home."

"I'd be sharing that cab."

We laugh weakly.

Fred stops by to present my outpatient treatment plan. "Heard you had a hissy fit this morning," he says.

"Yes, I did." And I explain why.

He gives me a discharge treatment plan containing the suggestions my counselor Gary made in my one-on-one session.

"The first thing you need to do is get some continuing help for your PTSD."

I disagree. "The first thing I need to do is get my diet straightened out. Getting my food cravings and blood sugar under control is critical for me."

We review other things—the writing class I will take, exercise.

He has an interesting observation: "Everything you've mentioned so far you're doing by yourself."

He's right. I need to do something about that—to see friends more often, seek out new friends.

I talk about the videos I've seen during the past ten days and how I'd like my husband to see them to understand my problem.

For the first time in a long time, I have a vision of the future and my husband is in it. And it makes me happy.

Fred mentions fun. I tell him I know that fun and joy do not exist in my life to any great extent. I resolve to work on that, too. I need to spend some more time with my "fun" friends.

As I talk with Fred, I realize that I feel lighter. Different. Huh! Is it just that all my Duffys are over?

I sign my treatment plan. Fred gives me a copy.

The doctor stops in again, and this time I'm able to speak with him. He reviews my test results once more.

My son Mike calls. We talk about our mutual admiration—how proud we are of each other. I tell him I did a great job raising him, and he tells me half-jokingly he was just thinking the same thing. This makes me feel wonderful. Mike is happy and at peace with himself.

Craig calls too. He has been a tremendous support to me, calling me nearly every day. Giving me kudos, helping lift my spirit.

Dinner is announced—cod, rice, fresh asparagus, apple crisp for dessert. I sit at a table with four other women and Robert. I ask Sharon, who, like me, is going home tomorrow, what we'll be talking about tomorrow night this time.

"Same thing: body products and physical symptoms," she replies.

We talk about the evening's upcoming movie, "28 Days". Sandra Bullock plays a woman going through a 28-day rehab program in place of jail time. I've never heard of the movie, but some of the women have seen it and we all decide to attend.

We all decide to attend!

I grab a cup of tea, head for the movie. Sandra Bullock is certain she doesn't belong in rehab. She mocks the place and does whatever she can to sabotage her stay, until she is threatened with being kicked out and sent to jail. Somewhere along the line, she realizes she truly does have a problem, and she faces it. It's a good movie. Even if it wasn't, I would have stayed—it felt good to be part of the group!

After the movie, I call Gary. We plan Sunday after I'm discharged. I want to go to Costco. I like to cook, and I need to get on track right away.

"Are you sure you're up to walking around Costco?" he wants to know.

Well, I've done nothing physical here except exercise my internal organs. I feel weak and atrophied. What better way to build up strength than by grocery shopping, hauling those 20-pound bags and boxes?

"Yes!" I respond enthusiastically.

Bedtime. I turn out the light, repeat some affirmations:

"I love living alcohol free."

"I drink only nonalcoholic beverages."

"Each day I get mentally and physically stronger."

DAY TEN

6 a.m. What a difference a day makes! My Duffys are done. I have my last rehab interview today, and then I'm going home!

It's my last day!

Well, except for two recap weekends—which, like Scarlett O'Hara, I'll think about tomorrow.

My vitals are 97.2, 91/57, 81. Weight 160. I've lost 5 pounds overall.

My rehab interview is scheduled for 8:30. I'm starving, but I can't eat.

Chet's door opens and he practically jogs past my door, singing. He backs up, pokes his head in to my doorway.

"I've been up since 4:30, I'm so pumped to be leaving." Continues his strut to the nurses' station.

I'm giddy. I open my curtains to feel the day. In the hall, I exchange phone numbers, e-mail addresses, and promises to keep in touch with Chet, Myra, and Sharon.

I'm brought in for my last sedation interview.

Before I go under, I tell Judy about my alcohol dream and how this scares me.

"It's perfectly normal," she says. "You may have them for years to come. They don't mean anything."

I'm glad it's normal, but I hope I don't have any more dreams like that. I don't want to spend another minute thinking about, acting, or reacting to alcohol!

I've made a couple of new affirmations for today. I begin

reading them and, as usual, wake up when the rehabilitation interview is over.

The results show I've reached a level 10 on the counter-conditioning scale. This interview concentrated mostly on what I will do when I get out, if I plan on following through with the treatment plan (yes), if I will call them if I get into trouble (yes).

Yes, yes, yes, and yes! Just let me the hell out of here!

It's 10:30. I ask for my clothes, but I can't have them yet—I have to be here for six more hours until the effect of my sedation drug wears off. So I relax, half dozing until lunch.

At lunch this last day—*this last day*—I sit with Chet and Sharon and we talk about our experience here. I can't believe all the things that came up for me: memories once submerged, now up and out. Emotions deliberately buried in a younger, more painful lifetime now hovering near the surface, waiting to be dealt with by the person I've become, am becoming.

We talk about what a roller coaster it's been—one day physically and emotionally exhausting, the next day incredibly relaxing. We could always tell who was having what treatment by the way they (we) walked, talked. Duffy days found us with our heads down, moving at slow speeds, frequently noncommunicative until afterward. Rehab interview days found us looking up and out, smiling, more sociable.

We again share some of our dreams now that we're alcohol free. I want to prepare for a new career. I want to stay alcohol free forever. I want to have fun. I want to regain the trust of my family and friends.

Back in my room, I'm given my clothes and overnight bag. I'm packing when Judy comes in to give me copies of all four sedation interviews. She also gives me her card and tells me to call her if I ever need to speak with anyone. I tell her I feel very comfortable with her and that if I need help, I will call.

We hug.

I remove the hospital ID bracelet with the "A" for alcoholic and put it in my packet to take home with me as another reminder.

On my way out, Fred gives me a round gold key chain with two-thirds of the inside circle missing. It has what looks like a purple and red butterfly on the front with the words "Only Takes One Perso", the rest of the words missing. On the back is a portion of the Serenity Prayer.

I'll get the second piece at my first recap, the last at my final recap. I'm so proud of this key chain. I worked hard to earn it.

Fred shakes my hand, wishes me luck.

As anxious as I am to leave, as grueling as this program was, I'll miss this place.

TWO WEEKS LATER: E-MAIL TO DR. SMITH, CHIEF OF STAFF OF SCHICK SHADEL HOSPITAL

Hi Dr. Smith,

My name is Kathleen S and I was discharged two weeks ago.

My first question may sound a little weird, but it is real: Why do I feel so good mentally? I'm not just talking about the absence of alcohol—in the past, I gave up alcohol for three months, six months, even two years, and I didn't feel the way I do now. Please let me explain:

My life has been going 'round in a futile circle for years

now, even through my periods of sobriety. I was always a goal-oriented person, yet for the past six years, I had no passions, no interests, got little joy from life. I drank, sobered up for a few weeks, drank again. All my energy revolved around alcohol, whether using it or not.

That hopeless circle has been broken in a big way. I have no cravings for alcohol at all. I don't even think about it. I changed my schedule to work fewer hours, enrolled in an educational program on the east coast that will train me to work as a nutrition consultant, made amends with my family, and generally have the most positive attitude towards life and living I've ever had.

What did it? Of course I realize none of this would be possible without the absence of alcohol, but there's something more. I'm thinking the rehab interviews played a big role, particularly the affirmations. But I don't know.

Can you tell me?

My second question involves the lectures you gave. While a patient there, I kept a very detailed journal, which I've decided to turn into a book.

It has evolved to include:

- The journal, recounting my personal experience in the program
- Some of the tools we were given: the consequences card for relapse prevention, how to create and use affirmations, some nutrition information, etc.
- I would also like to include some of the latest research on the medical aspects of addiction and treatment—excerpts from your three lectures (giving you the proper credit, of course). My daughter attended these with me and I know she was changed by it, particularly the one on

genetics. I'm sure you've published your research. Do you have reprints I might use to glean the information I'd want to use?

Dr. Smith, I can't thank you and the rest of Schick Shadel enough for living up to your promise: "Give us ten days and we'll give you back your life..." I have my life back. In fact, when I asked my daughter when the last time she saw me this enthusiastic about anything was, she thought a moment and then answered: "Never".

My husband is grateful and so are my other kids. In fact, my daughter and a son (20 and 25) will be illustrating the book. My other son (age 27) will be setting up a Web site for me.

You have given us a precious gift and for that you have our profound gratitude.

Sincerely,

Kathleen S

DR. SMITH'S RESPONSE THE NEXT DAY

I am very happy that you are feeling so good. I think that much of it is the lack of craving. I also think that part of it might be the affirmations.

I think that writing a book about your experience here would help other people (which is an additional way to make you feel good). Of course you can use any material I used in my lectures. However those were not my experiments. They were done by other researchers. I am just in the process of recording the lectures (on DVD) and they will be available soon if you want to use them in any way.

James W. Smith M.D.

30-DAY RECAP

This weekend I'm in a semi-private room. My roommate had a sedation interview this morning and has to hang around for a few hours before leaving. She left the room to give me some privacy.

I actually looked forward to coming here this morning—thought it would feel comfortable, a little like coming home.

But it doesn't.

I don't belong here anymore, and I want to leave. The only time I've thought about alcohol at all over these past 30 days is when I worked on my book, and now today thinking about my treatment.

Recaps require an overnight stay. One day you get a Duffy, one day you get a relaxation interview. You choose the order. I opted to have my Duffy treatment first. Get it over with.

Diane is again my nurse and greets me warmly. This must be the rewarding part of her job. You can't come for a recap if you've drunk at all during the past 30 days. So whoever shows up is doing well!

She tells me there will be a lot of glasses to drink, just like the last treatment. I get down parts of only two and can't drink anymore. My mouth won't open. I won't, can't drink anymore.

I throw up often and forcefully.

I don't have to finish—my continuing extreme revulsion is apparent. When there's a pause, Diane walks me back to my room. I have to stop halfway to breathe deeply so I won't throw up.

"It's only a few more steps," she says gently.

I take a few more steps and can't go any farther. She lets go of my arm, races into a room, and brings back a garbage can just in time for me to throw up into it, right there in the hallway.

We finally get to my room.

I'm already exhausted, and the three hours have just begun. She puts the gin-soaked rag next to my pillow. As soon as she leaves, I sweep it to the floor. I don't want to be sick anymore. And contrary to the rules, I don't think about my addiction, I don't need to. I fall asleep; I wake up each time they come in to take my pulse and ask my nausea level, but mostly I'm asleep.

The treatment ends.

I'm not in a socializing mood.

When I was admitted, I saw two familiar faces: one was Sharon's, and she was leaving. She said she's doing great—no cravings, no slips.

The other familiar face was Barbara's, who was the first patient I met (the one having Faradics treatment) when I was here for my 10-day stay. Barbara has relapsed and is here for a "six-pack", a shortened version of the 10-day program: three Faradics and three sedation interviews. I feel bad that she relapsed, but she seems accepting. And on the positive side, she's here getting help.

I don't even feel like writing in my journal. I watch television, read a little, talk on the phone to my kids and go to sleep.

Todd is conducting my sedation interview. I created a new list of affirmations and give it to him to key in to the computer.

He returns it to me, and once again I read and drift off. The results show I have an alcohol aversion level of 11 on a scale of 1 to 10!

Other results:

Question: Do you have difficulty being around people who drink or use other drugs?
Answer: No.

Question: Do you have any difficulty staying alcohol and drug free?
Answer: No.

Question: Do you have any negative feelings about staying sober?
Answer: No.

Question: Now that you're sober, what is great in your life?
Answer: I have come to an understanding about my job; I am reconciling with my husband; my kids and I have a great relationship; and I will be taking classes on nutrition and holistic health.

Question: How's your self-esteem and self-confidence?
Answer: Pretty good.

I can't wait to get out of here.

On my way out, I'm given a key chain with two-thirds of the inner circle complete: "Only Takes One Person to Change Your Life-" on the front, more of the Serenity Prayer on the back.

90-DAY RECAP

I want to be here this time even less than I did for the 30-day recap. I decide to have my sedation interview first, my Duffy the second day, but I realize I really don't want to do the Duffy at all. I still have no cravings, and I don't think about alcohol except when I'm here.

The doctor says the patient knows best, so I waive my Duffy rights. A nurse comes in and asks me to confirm my request. I do.

I hope I've done the right thing and didn't just chicken out.

I have my sedation interview. I've prepared 24 new affirmations. Judy is conducting the interview. She's good for me—she tells me my affirmations are always perfect for the stage I'm at. I read a few and then "zzzzzzzzzzz…".

She tells me I literally slept through most of it, and they had to keep prodding me to wake up. But my aversion level is still over 10.

A few hours later, I'm discharged.

I am a graduate, and I take a sticker for my memories. I get the third, completed key ring. It has the whole Serenity Prayer on one side, and on the other the completed message: "It Only Takes One Person to Change Your Life—You".

How true that is.

I'm feeling good from my head to my shoes,
Know where I'm goin' and I know what to do,
I tidied up my point of view,
I got a new attitude!

New Attitude
Jon Gilutin, Bunny Hull, Sharon Terea Robinson

PART 3
AFTER

ME—FIVE YEARS LATER!

Five years have passed. Five years!

When I first got out I was worried about having too much time on my hands—unstructured time was one of my many triggers. So I made myself my priority. I vowed to get better physically, mentally, emotionally.

Physically, those drinking years took their toll. I didn't bounce back the way I thought I would, should, when I stopped drinking. I decided to find out why and do something about it.

I enrolled in a year-long nutrition and health coaching program and I became my first client! I concentrated on improving my digestive system—the reflux, bloating, the mood swings (yes, these can be caused by digestive "stuff"), the allergies. At 61 (okay, 61 and a half!) I feel better physically and have more energy than I've had since my twenties.

Emotionally, writing this book was therapeutic. I was amazed to learn during treatment just how much my feelings were still rooted in the past, how those scars stood in my way. I spent time confronting my ghosts. They are gradually losing power over me.

I had never dealt with my brothers' deaths, never grieved because I was so angry. But after treatment I was able to mourn their lives, which they lost long before they stopped breathing. I talk to them now and then and keep them in my thoughts.

I probably will always have mixed feelings about my father. I do believe he loved me. I understand he had a disease. I know his generation often thought of beatings as an acceptable form of discipline. But the physical abuse: feeling his belt myself, seeing Mike's pain as he got beaten, are things I can't easily forget.

It's still hard to completely forgive the emotional abuse, but I no longer harbor anger or hatred towards him. And I talk to him once in awhile too, mostly with a smile on my face. I remember more and more about how funny he could be when sober, how he would break into song for no reason (a trait which I've inherited, much to the chagrin of my friends and family!), how handsome he was.

For all of them—my father and two brothers—there is sorrow. Sorrow that they were unable to get the help they desperately needed, when they needed it. Sorrow for what could have been, but wasn't.

I love my mother fiercely, and "forgive" her for the decisions she made within the context of her own life and circumstances, as if that power is really mine to give. Perhaps a better way of saying it is that I am more accepting, less judgmental, and I no longer feel anger towards her.

She is 90, in failing health, and when she is gone I will be devastated.

She heard I wrote a book but has not expressed an interest in reading it (although other family members, including my one remaining brother, have read it). I do believe she would be hurt by the book, seeing events through my eyes. I don't need to go there.

My mother and I are very close. And remember how hard it was for her to say "I love you"? Not a phone call ends these days without each of us saying those words to each other. And often she says it first! Things really can change…

I'm a grandma to two little boys (from my son Mike), who at this writing are one and three years old. They bring me joy. Pure joy. I'm struggling with the fact that I live across the country from them – I want to be part of the village that raises them.

My husband and I are still together. I don't drink any more, and he doesn't belittle me. Do we still have issues? Of course. But we are still working on stuff, probably always will be.

Gary retired a few months ago and that's been an adjustment for both of us, since I need to work a few more years. I'm still at the same place, although my job has changed. I have more responsibility. It's stressful sometimes, but good.

A few months after the first edition of my book was published, I gave a copy to the woman who was my manager at the time I was treated. I thanked her for being so supportive, even when she didn't know what my problem was. She and I have become really good friends.

I continue to create goals: writing this book was one of them. But my goal to be on Oprah with it? Well—I wrote to her show but they weren't interested. Neither were Ellen, David Letterman, Dr. Phil, or any of the local Seattle stations. Huh! With my fifth anniversary edition, maybe I'll try "The View".

I still use affirmations periodically, when I want to change or create something in my life. In fact, I started a new list this week. I keep it next to the sink, see it first thing in the morning and last thing at night. I strongly believe in the power of self-talk.

Another dream I realized is that for three years now, every other Sunday I give a talk to Schick patients on nutrition, specifically low blood sugar and cravings. It is so gratifying when people begin to understand how important their diet is to their health, well-being and continued abstinence. A plan for improved nutrition should be part of everyone's relapse prevention kit, no matter what treatment program they're going through.

A few years ago I started a chemical dependency certification (CDP) program to get more involved in counseling. I took about half the credits and stopped going.

The program was good, but also frustrating and a little depressing. I have a degree in public health, where the emphasis is on outcomes. What works? Is there a significant difference in results between treatment A and treatment B?

There doesn't seem to be that kind of rigor in the field of addiction. There doesn't appear to be a standard definition or measurement of treatment success. How can we recommend specific programs if we don't know how successful they are for various types of addiction?

Maybe my energies would be better served elsewhere in the addiction field, I don't know. What I do know is that for the time being, I'm content doing wellness workshops at Schick.

All in all, when I look back at these five years I think "Wow! If I had been drinking, I wouldn't have done any of this." The truth is I might not even be alive.

I probably *wouldn't* be alive...

The best news is: I have thoughts of alcohol sometimes, I may occasionally dream of it, but I continue to have no cravings. Five years and I continue to have no cravings!

I can be around people who are drinking. Neither the

sight nor the smell make me want to drink. On the other hand, I don't get nauseous around alcohol either.

What else has happened? Well, the sneaky, secretive side of me that knew how to lie so convincingly (I could've won an Academy Award!) is gone. I've got nothing to hide. And *that* feels good!

I still have issues with just being, and with having fun. But I try.

I want to say one more thing about alcoholism. Since I accepted addiction as a disease, I also had to accept that I couldn't be "cured", that there is no cure, at least not yet. I can be alcohol's slave again in a very short time simply by reintroducing the substance into my life. I know and accept this.

So I no longer say: "I used to be an alcoholic". What I say when I'm out with people I don't know well, people who are drinking and look to me for my order is: "I don't drink – I'll have water". What I say when I have to tell a doctor or other professional about my background is: "I'm an alcoholic but I gave up drinking years ago."

I have a disease. But like the commercial says: "it doesn't have me!"

Has everything been perfect in my life since I left Schick?

Please.

My son Craig told us about his cocaine and alcohol problem about a year after I graduated from Schick. For anyone who has a child with an addiction, you know how devastating this is, how helpless you feel as a parent.

But there was more pain to come: when he came back from treatment, he had a lot of anger towards my husband and me for some significant miscommunication. Misunderstandings on both sides over what he was going through. He didn't speak to us for a year and a half. It was one of the most painful experiences of my life—it was as if he died, so abruptly and completely did he cut us out of his life.

My husband was diagnosed with bladder cancer about three years ago and has since had two surgeries and chemotherapy. He has to have a checkup every three months. Yesterday he had his third cancer-free checkup in a row, for a total of nine months without the disease recurring.

It was Gary's cancer that brought our family back together. Craig was able to talk things over with us, and the family was able to reconcile.

Craig has been clean for four years now, has gotten married to a talented, supportive woman, and has matured into a wonderful, wonderful man. I frequently tear up when talking with him – I am that proud.

In the past these things – my husband's cancer, my son's addiction and his severing our relationship – would have been enough to send me back to the bottle. But I didn't go there. With the tools and conditioning I was given at Schick, I was able to get through these life-changing events without drinking.

When I use the word miracle to describe my life now, I'm not exaggerating. My continued existence on this planet, with no cravings for alcohol, is nothing short of miraculous.

Now when I think about alcohol, my thoughts always follow through to what it was like waking up the next morning. Or rather, returning to consciousness the next day.

And to something else I've learned: we have something in our biochemistry that remembers where we were in our using career. We can never go back to the beginning when using might have been fun or produced a high. Because very shortly we will be exactly where we left off. We will need just as much substance to get us to where we think we want to go as if we'd never stopped. And we will be those same addicted creatures in a very, very short time. We can't control it. Ever. Thinking we can is delusional.

People who have relapsed tell me they were sober for four, ten, twelve years—I recently heard of someone clean for 40 years!—and thought they were at a point where they could control their use. And so they had a drink. Then two. Then they were back in treatment and had to learn all over again that they cannot drink or use. Period.

Is that unfair? Perhaps. But if you're really going to get on top of this disease, you have to accept it. Grieve if you must, for it is a loss, but accept it. It's never going to change.

Here's something that's really unfair. Terribly unfair: There are seven kids in the next generation of my family. At various times and in various circumstances, substance abuse has affected several of them.

I asked Craig if I could share the fact that he has an addiction, and he said yes. Other than him, I won't identify anyone else because their stories are their own to tell. Or not. But it is heartbreaking knowing that we are passing on this disease.

Please heed Dr. Smith's advice and talk to your kids often. And very, very candidly.

SCHICK SHADEL HOSPITAL
FIVE YEARS LATER

As I approach Schick Shadel Hospital this morning to do my nutrition workshop, I'm thinking about my five-year anniversary. I'm in a particularly good mood and I am particularly observant—thinking about the many changes that have taken place since I was here as a patient.

A beautiful rock garden greets you at the top of the driveway, the water from the fountain clear, fresh. I roll my windows down to hear the soothing sound of it cascading to the bottom. Walking paths have been designed around the perimeter of the property with benches placed here and there for enjoying the serenity.

I park my car, walk into the lobby. It has also been redone—beautiful tiled floors, fireplace, soft lighting. Very welcoming. Very soothing.

The patients look different too. Men and women alike outfitted in sharp, teal "scrubs" —the power suit of the day. Their rooms have been remodeled—hardwood floors, fireplaces, new beds, soft colors. And Wi-Fi!

One fun fact I've learned is that many patients plan their recaps with their roommates or others they've gotten to know while here. Once, there was a group of ten that came back together at 30 days to give each other support!

I recognize some of the staff: There's Diane and Debbie… Still doing their jobs with compassion and humor.

And did I mention salad bar?

Dr. Smith, Medical Director of the Hospital, died several years ago. What a special man. I attended his memorial service, as did hundreds of people—many former patients, many distinguished colleagues. Dr. Smith was at Schick Shadel for more than 45 years, and is still missed. More than just memories have survived him, however. His lectures were put on DVD before he died, so patients can still learn from him.

Dr. Davis is the new Medical Director. They've also hired a full-time Research Director, Dr. Elkins. Please read the afterword Dr. Elkins wrote to get an idea of the ground-breaking addiction research being conducted at Schick.

The counseling program has undergone significant changes with the addition of staff and the reorganization of workshops. Paula Fisher is the Director of Counseling, with Jerome Walters as Program Director.

Every day there are at least five classes a patient can attend, with topics ranging from setting goals, the genetics of addiction, being less judgmental about yourself and others, building confidence, grief and loss, no-regret living, etc.

I've attended many of these in the past few months because they are so important, targeted, and because as always, I'm a work in progress —there's always something to learn.

The patient population at Schick has changed as well. These days they are treating more than 1,000 patients a year and have started doing Duffy treatments for prescription drugs.

I've learned that Schick Shadel patients are not court mandated, which means every one of them is here voluntarily. That the Hospital's census levels are consistently high, that the Hospital has the lowest number of patients checking out against medical advice (AMA) in the industry speaks volumes about the treatment. It answers some critics' claims that counter-conditioning therapy is sadistic. Patients are voluntarily choosing Schick, and voluntarily seeing their treatment through to the end, more so than any other program.

If I sound like a commercial for Schick, I don't apologize. I'm amazed at how much misinformation, prejudice, and resistance exists out there. We should be grateful we have options. There is no one "right" way to get clean.

I have nothing against any of the things I tried on my road to recovery, including AA. They just didn't work for me. And while I don't attend, the fellowship and support of AA meetings and related groups like AlAnon are invaluable for many, many people. If you need the support, the community, the fellowship—please, please attend.

But please, please be aware that there are other avenues to sobriety, other combinations of treatment and support. Let's embrace these options.

Does Schick work for everyone? Of course not. *Nothing works for everyone!* But it does work for a lot of people. And while there appears to be no industry standard for measuring success, Schick considers treatment successful if the patient is clean and sober one year after completion of the program. With that as the measure, their success rate for alcohol is around 70%. That is very, very high.

DIFFERENT STROKES FOR DIFFERENT FOLKS...

Your road to recovery is as unique as your path to addiction. What works for one does not necessarily work for others.

When I think of how I almost didn't come to Schick

Shadel because of my counselor's comments, it makes me sad. And angry. If I hadn't had the confidence, I would've heeded her advice. And I don't know where I'd be today.

Other people have expressed doubts in the humanity, the ethics of this treatment, as if Schick Shadel is the same institution that employed Nurse Ratchet in "One Flew Over the Cuckoo's Nest". I hope my story will help put those doubts to rest.

Was the treatment hard?

Yes. The five Duffy treatments were hard.

Compared to a lifetime of addiction?

No contest.

And isn't that the bottom line?

A NOTE FROM THE AUTHOR

This book, originally published under the title: "Drink Up! A Recovery Road Less Traveled", was revised and retitled to celebrate my five-year alcohol-free anniversary.

One of the most rewarding things about writing and publishing the book has been hearing from the people who read it. Many tell me they give the book to one or two other people so their loved ones can understand what they are going through, both with the disease, and with the treatment.

Where are you in the world, in your life, and how did you come to be reading this book? I'd love to hear from you. Can you take a minute and email me at:

kathleens@recoveru.com

to say hello? I respond to all emails.

Thank you for reading my story and I wish you the very, very best.

Kathleen S

A Recovery Road Less Traveled...

Two roads diverged in a wood, and I-
I took the one less traveled by
And that has made all the difference

Robert Frost
"The Road Not Taken"

DEDICATION

This book is dedicated to the staff of Schick Shadel Hospital, particularly Diane, Debbie, Dr. Smith, and to the Hospital owners, all of whom are former patients who stepped in to buy the Hospital in 2002 when its future was in doubt. They bought it in part because they wanted this treatment available if addiction appeared in subsequent generations of their own families.

Thank you.
Kathleen S

AFTERWORD

Our hospital, originally called Shadel Hospital, was started by Charles Shadel in 1935 (author's note: coincidentally the same year AA was founded) and began as an alcoholism treatment program only. In 1960 while in Family Practice, I was asked to be a part-time Medical Director to replace the existing part-time Medical Director who, because of ill health, was forced to retire.

At that time I did not have a favorable attitude toward alcoholics but agreed to fill in "temporarily" until a more interested director could be found. Fortunately, I quickly learned that alcoholics were just like other people with a disease from which most of them would recover with the proper treatment. At Shadel Hospital we saved many lives and families. I found this to be extremely emotionally rewarding, so rewarding that I gave up my private family practice and began working full time in addiction medicine.

In 1964, J. Patrick Frawley Jr., the person who developed the Paper Mate Pen and was at the time chairman of Schick Safety Razor Company, treated at Shadel for alcoholism. He was so impressed with what happened to him that he bought the Hospital (that is why the present name is Schick Shadel Hospital) and spent 6 million dollars researching habit formation. In the process we developed treatments for tobacco smoking and for addictions to cocaine, methamphetamine, marijuana and narcotics.

I am glad that one of our patients, Kathleen S, wrote a book about the treatment from the patient's perspective. This book is written factually, with warmth and humor. I hope it will encourage others to give up their addiction and regain their lives again.

James W. Smith, M.D.
Chief of Staff
Schick Shadel Hospital
Seattle, Washington
August, 2005

AFTERWORD

I was given a copy of Kathleen S's excellent book: *"Drink Up! – A Recovery Road Less Traveled"* shortly after arriving in Seattle in 2008 as Schick Shadel Hospital's first full-time Research Director. I thoroughly enjoyed Kathy's frank and personalized description of her treatment experiences; she successfully captured the supportive social milieu and the unique treatments that empower the recoveries of Schick Shadel's patients. Her book is well-written, moving, and even humorous at times.

This update includes new content and insights from her broadened perspective following five years of sobriety. Kathy's words and her typically excellent outcome will encourage others who can benefit from walking in her footsteps.

A PREVIEW OF SCHICK SHADEL HOSPITAL'S CURRENT RESEARCH PROJECT...

We are doing some amazing research at Schick, which Kathy asked me to preview here. During my career, I have been able to objectively confirm via physiological and behavioral evidence that nausea-based counter-conditioning therapy actually produces profound and long-lasting conditioned aversions to the sight, smell, taste, and frequently to the mere thought of the targeted addictive substances. These studies also revealed that nausea-based, counter-conditioning therapy, which capitalizes on the ancient and highly protective process of taste aversion learning, also totally eliminates the persistent substance cravings that taint the early recoveries of most alcoholics who achieve sobriety without the brain altering benefits of counter conditioning therapy. This accounts for the comfortable abstinence of Schick Shadel's patients who have been liberated from "white knuckled" cravings.

Several scientists recently have shown that the new brain scan technologies (i.e., PET scan and fMRI neuroimaging) can detect localized brain activations in conscious addicted individuals who are actively craving their problem substance(s). University of Washington scientists and I will extend these findings by neuroimaging the brain activation transformations that underlie the counter conditioning (Duffy) produced transition from substance-induced cravings to substance-induced aversions.

We hypothesize that the Duffy treatments will eliminate the localized brain activations that subserve cravings just as they eliminate the cravings themselves. We additionally predict that, following successful Duffy conditioning, the banished brain cravings activations will be replaced by a new brain activation pattern that is indicative of counter conditioned rejection responses on the part of patients who are presented with or reminded of their problem substance(s). These findings would powerfully support the disease concept of addiction by showing that our Duffy treatments replace pathological brain activated indices of substance cravings with abstinence promoting brain activated indices of substance aversions. The expected localized brain activation indices of the Duffy-induced counter conditioned aversions should more precisely define the involved brain regions.

I thank Kathy for the opportunity to preview these exciting prospects, and to explicate their positive implications for widespread acceptance of Schick Shadel's unique anti-cravings treatment. The neuroimaging findings and other research results will be described and referenced on the Hospital Web Site at www.schickshadel.com.

Ralph L. Elkins, Ph.D.
Research Director
Schick Shadel Hospital

APPENDIX

Here is the complete list (in alphabetical order) of throw-up synonyms I collected:

Barf	Heave
Be sick	Hug the porcelain bowl
Belch	Hurl
Blow Chunks	Puke
Boot	Purge
Buick????	Ralf
Call Ralph	Regurgitate
Cast	Retch
Cat	Rolf
Chuck	Spew
Discharge	Toss
Disgorge	Toss my cookies
Eject	Upchuck
Gag	Vomit
Gush	Zak
Honk	Zook

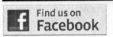

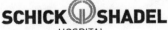